D1357599

Modeling Public Health
and Healthcare Systems

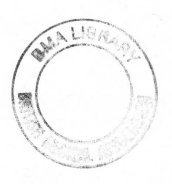

Modeling Public Health and Healthcare Systems

Sanjay Basu, MD, PhD

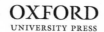

OXFORD
UNIVERSITY PRESS

OXFORD
UNIVERSITY PRESS

Oxford University Press is a department of the University of Oxford. It furthers the University's objective of excellence in research, scholarship, and education by publishing worldwide. Oxford is a registered trade mark of Oxford University Press in the UK and certain other countries.

Published in the United States of America by Oxford University Press
198 Madison Avenue, New York, NY 10016, United States of America.

© Oxford University Press 2018

Library of Congress Cataloging-in-Publication Data
Names: Basu, Sanjay, 1980– author.
Title: Modeling public health and healthcare systems / Sanjay Basu.
Description: Oxford ; New York : Oxford University Press, [2018] |
Includes bibliographical references and index.
Identifiers: LCCN 2017021099 | ISBN 9780190667924 (hardback : alk. paper)
Subjects: | MESH: Public Health—statistics & numerical data |
Models, Statistical | Delivery of Health Care—statistics &
numerical data | Computer Simulation
Classification: LCC RA409 | NLM WA 950 | DDC 362.1072/7—dc23
LC record available at https://lccn.loc.gov/2017021099

This material is not intended to be, and should not be considered, a substitute for medical or other professional advice. Treatment for the conditions described in this material is highly dependent on the individual circumstances. And, while this material is designed to offer accurate information with respect to the subject matter covered and to be current as of the time it was written, research and knowledge about medical and health issues is constantly evolving and dose schedules for medications are being revised continually, with new side effects recognized and accounted for regularly. Readers must therefore always check the product information and clinical procedures with the most up-to-date published product information and data sheets provided by the manufacturers and the most recent codes of conduct and safety regulation. The publisher and the authors make no representations or warranties to readers, express or implied, as to the accuracy or completeness of this material. Without limiting the foregoing, the publisher and the authors make no representations or warranties as to the accuracy or efficacy of the drug dosages mentioned in the material. The authors and the publisher do not accept, and expressly disclaim, any responsibility for any liability, loss or risk that may be claimed or incurred as a consequence of the use and/or application of any of the contents of this material.

1 3 5 7 9 8 6 4 2

Printed by Sheridan Books, Inc., United States of America

CONTENTS

INTRODUCTION

KNOWING WHERE TO MARK THE "X"

In the early 20th century, a bearded gnome was sighted by the children of Schenectady, New York. The gnome, they claimed, would row along Schenectady's waterways in a canoe. The gnome was often sighted smoking a panatela cigar while leaning over a tiny desk positioned in the bottom of the canoe, on which he scribbling intently. The gnome's young followers sometimes collected papers that flew out of the boat and into the water as evidence to present to their disbelieving parents.

Outside the city, the gnome had become well-known to scientists—including Thomas Edison, Albert Einstein, and Nicola Tesla—who referred to him as "The Little Giant of Schenectady." Among the scientific community, the four-foot-tall man, Charles Steinmetz, was amongst the world's most talented electrical engineers. He suffered from short stature due to a genetic disease known as kyphosis, but—despite skepticism from the city's children—had obtained a position among the elite engineering team at the General Electric Company of Schenectady.

Steinmetz was not only known for deriving differential equations while drifting on his canoe, but also for collecting Gila monsters, alligators, and rattlesnakes, which he tended to in a customized mansion that sat atop one of the city's popular avenues. Though eccentric, Steinmetz secured his role in the history of American innovation by carefully dissecting the period's toughest engineering problems and delivering solutions critical to the future of industry. He had, for instance, devised a mathematical law known as the Law of Hysteresis (or Steinmetz's Law), which explained how energy dissipates through heat, thus paving the way for more efficient electrical power generators.

But Steinmetz's image as an innovator in the American popular parlance did not solidify until an edition of *Life Magazine* in 1965 revealed his interactions with the industrial magnate Henry Ford, who operated a large automobile factory in Dearborn, Michigan. Steinmetz was invited by Ford to his factory, which was experiencing a perplexing problem with a massive electrical power generator. Steinmetz had been told that Ford's engineering team could not decipher how to fix the generator despite multiple attempts to modify it. Apparently, the team disagreed about what to do. Some engineers on the team wanting to replace expensive parts of the machine's backbone. Others wanted to continue adding patches as bandages to the generator's periphery in a desperate trial-and-error attempt to get the machine working as soon as possible.

According to legend, Steinmetz arrived in Dearborn and dismissed all of Ford's engineers, ignoring their theories and proposals. He demanded a notebook and a pencil. In isolation, he mentally diagnosed the machine's ailments without opening a single panel of the massive metal structure. He listened to its wounded whirring, slept next to the machine in a cot, and jotted down notes for two days and two nights. He carefully diagrammed the machine and its parts, tracing every component of its infrastructure and every step required to operate it. At the end of the second night, he apparently left the factory to purchase a piece of chalk and returned to request a ladder, which he used to climb aboard the generator and mark a large chalk "X" on one of the machine's main panels. He instructed Ford's engineering team to remove the panel at the location of the "X" and replace 16 turns of copper wire from a coil underneath. Steinmetz's instructions were followed incredulously by the Ford engineering team, but the generator restarted in perfect working order.

Steinmetz had relieved Henry Ford of a major dilemma. He was asked by Ford to mail a bill for his consulting services. Steinmetz sent Ford a request for $10,000— approximately $208 per hour for two days' work. In disbelief, Steinmetz was asked by the accountants at Ford's company for an itemized invoice to justify the expense, to which Steinmetz replied:

Making chalk mark on generator $1
Knowing where to make mark $9,999

Steinmetz was paid in full.[1]

WHAT DO WE MEAN BY "MODELING" PUBLIC HEALTH AND HEALTHCARE SYSTEMS?

The legend of Charles Steinmetz offers a lesson for those of us concerned with modern public health and healthcare systems. Many of the daily challenges faced in the public health and healthcare sectors are complex "operational" problems—dilemmas that involve systems that are at least as convoluted as Henry Ford's generator, if not more so. People working in the public health and healthcare fields commonly face problems with ineffective or "broken" operational environments. These environments lead to questions such as: "Why are patients waiting so long in the emergency department before being seen by a doctor?", "Why are we still seeing cases of an infectious disease in our community despite a massive vaccination program that was supposed to have eradicated it?", or "Why are we paying so much for this new laboratory test instead of using a cheaper alternative?"

When faced with public health or healthcare delivery problems, many people respond with the same desperation as Ford's engineers: either wanting to replace expensive, fundamental parts of a complex system ("Fire the current doctor, hire a new one, and hopefully the waiting times in the emergency department will be reduced"). Others simply add patches as superficial bandages that are unlikely to fix the underlying dilemma ("Start an education program to inform patients about when the emergency department is busiest so they'll come at another time"—a suggestion I received when consulting for a local hospital).

As an alternative to using a desperate trial-and-error approach, we can learn from Steinmetz's strategy: to carefully diagram the key components of the complex problem we are attempting to solve. We can analyze each element of the diagram systematically until we identify the root cause of the problem. The method of carefully diagramming a problem is what we now call "modeling." Modeling involves creating an abstract model of a real-world problem to help us diagnose and treat the problem in a thoughtful, systematic, and meticulous way. Unlike Steinmetz, we have the luxury of not simply using a notebook and pencil (though these tools are often adequate for many problems), but of also using modern high-performance computers to assist us in creating and analyzing our models.

Our goal in this book is to teach students "where to put the X" on major healthcare and public health problems that involve breakdowns and failures in our systems. These breakdowns and failures produce long waiting lines, poorly distributed human or material resources, and poorly conceived plans for how to diagnose the neediest patients or provide them with the best treatment. Many of these problems have been extensively studied through Steinmetz's approach of modeling a problem. The modeling field has identified several effective strategies for solving common problems in public health and healthcare delivery. In this book, we present these common strategies through a case-based approach to sequentially build students' skills for "knowing where to mark the X."

EXAMPLES OF THE TYPES OF PROBLEMS WE'LL LEARN HOW TO SOLVE

This book teaches both traditional and newer modeling strategies through a series of practice problems. The book's aim is to empower students to learn how to develop and apply models by working through the model development process, motivated by real-world problems. Critically, the book is aimed at teaching students common "templates" for solving different kinds of problems and providing classical equations that allow us to see how they can be generalized to a wide range of circumstances.

The book's format for solving problems can best be illustrated through a few specific examples.

Example Problem 1: Testing for Alzheimer's

A new test has been devised for Alzheimer's disease by Canadian researchers at the University of Alberta using saliva to test whether patients are experiencing the early stages of Alzheimer's disease. The laboratory director at the University has purchased equipment to offer patients the new test but is facing an irritating (and common) problem: the laboratory equipment to perform the test is imperfect. In this case, the equipment can run the new test properly on 80% of the samples but fails to run the test properly on the other 20% (note that we have used simplified numbers in these examples; these numbers should not be taken as "real" performance data). Those 20% of samples that fail to run properly are ruined in the testing process, so the laboratory director has to call a physician to find the patient and collect an entirely new sample to process the 20% of samples over again. Even worse, the equipment still generates costs for all samples put into the machine, even if the test fails to run properly. Every sample put into the machine (even the 20% that failed to run properly) costs about $100 each, due to material and personnel costs.

An enterprising laboratory company salesperson has contacted the laboratory director with an offer: suppose the salesperson could provide the laboratory with a new piece of equipment that can run the test properly on 90% of samples. The new equipment fails to run the test properly only 10% of the time (rather than 20% of the time), but costs $120 per sample to run due to the required material and personnel costs (rather than $100 per sample with the existing equipment).

The laboratory director had to decide: should she pay for the new piece of equipment or stick to the current cheaper, but less reliable, equipment?

Solution to Example Problem 1

This type of dilemma is known as a "value of information" problem, which is a type of problem in which we are paying for new information (in this case, a test result) and need to know how much we should be willing to pay for the new information. Value of information problems are common when we have to compare information from a traditional source (here, an old piece of equipment) with information from a new source with different characteristics, such as a different rate of reliability.

Value of information problems are typically solved by calculating the average (expected) cost of doing business under the status quo situation and comparing it to an estimate of the expected cost of doing business under the proposed new situation. In the status quo situation, the laboratory director must spend $100 per sample but recollect and reanalyze 20% of the samples. Figure I.1 illustrates the process of analyzing a patient's sample and reveals the (potentially infinitely long) process in which a sample can fail to run properly on the first try, then again fail to run properly on the second try, and so on. A sequence like this, in which each time point can result in success or failure leading to a potentially infinitely long sequence of events, is called a Bernoulli process.

Suppose we call the average expected cost of running each sample with the current status quo equipment variable E. We know that, 80% of the time, we expect the sample to run just fine the first try, we will pay $100 for it, and we'll be all done. But 20% of the time, we expect the sample to fail to run properly, we will pay $100 for the failed test, and we'll have to go back and start all over again, in which case the future will look like it did at the beginning of the process and we'll expect to pay another E dollars.

The expected cost of running each sample in the current status quo situation can be described by the following equation:

$$E = 0.8 \times \$100 + 0.2 \times (\$100 + E).$$ [Equation I.1]

If we rearrange the equation to solve for the value of E, we find that the current expected cost of running a sample with the status quo equipment, taking into account the risk of failure, is $E = \$125$ per sample.

Now we can compare this cost to the expected cost of running a sample using the new piece of equipment being offered by the salesperson. Suppose we call the average expected cost of running each sample with the new equipment variable F.

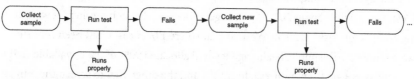

FIGURE I.1 **Example problem 1: Following a patient's laboratory sample as it undergoes testing.** After collecting a patient sample, some of the time the sample will run properly when put into the laboratory equipment, but a fraction of the time, the sample will fail to run properly, and we will pay for the failed test and restart the process by collecting a new sample. After a test fails, the future will look like it did at the beginning of the process, and the sequence of events could continue perpetually until a test is run successfully.

We were told that the new equipment costs $120 for each run but only fails 10% of the time (being successful 90% of the time). Therefore, the expected cost of running each sample with the new equipment can be described by the following equation:

$$F = 0.9 \times \$120 + 0.1 \times \left(\$120 + F\right).$$
[Equation I.2]

Solving this equation, we find that $F = \$133$ per sample.

In other words, the new test—although more reliable—is more expensive on average. Hence, if the laboratory director were making the decision about what equipment to use based on cost alone—not taking into account inconvenience or other important factors—the director would stick with the current equipment.

In Chapter 2, we'll explore several other scenarios for value of information problems, such as what price the laboratory director should negotiate before purchasing the new equipment to produce a net savings for her laboratory.

Example Problem 2: Screening for Ebola

In March 2014, several countries in West Africa experienced the largest-ever outbreak of the viral illness Ebola. Ebola can cause fever, severe diarrhea and vomiting, abdominal pain, headaches, and profound bruising and bleeding. More than 28,000 cases, resulting in at least 11,000 deaths, occurred from the March 2014 outbreak.[2] Because the disease is spread through bodily fluids, including sweat and saliva, many authorities were concerned about its transmission among travelers to and from the West African region. Flights in and out of airports were often delayed so that public health officials could ask travelers whether they were experiencing symptoms of the disease and to check their temperatures to detect anyone with a fever.

Unfortunately, as is typically the case, most public health agencies did not have sufficient personnel to screen every passenger at every major airport. At one major airport, for example, the national public health agency only had sufficient personnel available to screen 5% of people who traveled through the airport. About 80% of passengers traveling through the airport were from "low-risk" areas outside of West Africa, while about 20% of passengers traveling through the airport were coming from "high-risk" areas in West Africa, where Ebola cases had been reported in large numbers. The public health agency had allocated 90% of their available staff to screen passengers from high-risk locations and the other 10% to screen the remaining low-risk travelers.

A government official from the country wondered how likely it was for the country's under-staffed public health agency to be able to detect a case of Ebola at the airport. He asked public health agency officials: if a person is already infected with

Ebola but comes from a low risk area, what are the public health agency's chances of detecting the infected person?

Solution to Example Problem 2

This is an example of a typical screening problem, which involves calculating how much public health benefit might be achieved by searching a group of people for disease. To solve this type of problem, we typically start by estimating the "capture probability," or the chance of finding the person of interest if that person exists in the location we are screening. In this case, the capture probability is the probability of finding a person infected with Ebola if an infected person is in the airport.

To solve the problem, we can envision a simple diagram (Figure I.2) to help us picture the airport and the types of individuals being screened there.

In the diagram, we have drawn a typical set of 100 passengers in the airport under consideration. As stated in the problem, 20 of these passengers are from high-risk areas, and the other 80 are from low risk areas. The inner dashed rectangle shows our personnel resources available to conduct the screening exercise, with 90% of those resources devoted to the high-risk travelers and the other 10% to the low-risk travelers.

To answer the question of how likely we are to find an infected traveler from a low-risk area if such a traveler is passing through our airport, we can start by calculating what the maximum probability would be for finding such a traveler if all of our resources had been devoted to the low-risk group. In the scenario in which all of our

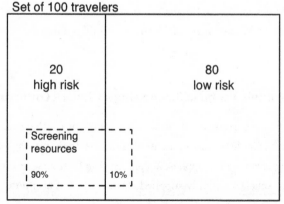

FIGURE I.2 Example problem 2: Screening travelers in an airport for Ebola symptoms. For every group of 100 travelers, 80 are from low risk areas, while 20 are from high risk areas. The local public health agency only has the personnel resources necessary to screen five of every 100 travelers, and has devoted 90% of these resources to screen travelers from high risk areas, with the other 10% screening traveling from low risk areas.

resources are devoted to the low-risk group, at most 5 of every 80 low-risk travelers would be screened. Hence, at most 5 of the 80, which equals 6.25%, is the chance that a low-risk traveler with Ebola would be caught by the screening program. But we only devoted 10% of our screening resources to screening the low-risk travelers; hence, our agency's chances of detecting the infected person from a low-risk area (the capture probability, abbreviated $p(capture)_{lowrisk}$) is:

$$p(capture)_{lowrisk} = 0.1 \times \frac{5}{80} = 0.6\%. \qquad \text{[Equation I.3]}$$

Analogously, we can ask the question of what the agency's chances are of detecting an infected person in the airport if that infected person is from a high-risk area. At most, if all resources were allocated to screening high-risk people, we could detect 5 of every 20 high-risk passengers, or 25%. But we devoted 90% rather than 100% of the screening resources to screening the high risk-travelers; hence, our agency's chances of detecting the infected person from a high risk area ($p(capture)_{highrisk}$) is:

$$p(capture)_{highrisk} = 0.9 \times \frac{5}{20} = 22.5\%. \qquad \text{[Equation I.4]}$$

Overall, these results are fairly depressing. Even if an infected traveler is coming from a high-risk area and we are devoting the vast majority of our resources to finding him, we still have less than a one in four chance of finding him before he jets off to a new area and potentially spreads the virus.

In Chapter 1, we will analyze more screening problems, particularly for cases where the screening method itself is not 100% accurate. We will also derive a strategy to determine what the "optimal allocation" of resources would be for any given screening problem to maximize our chances of finding a person with a disease of interest.

Example Problem 3: Stopping a Cholera Outbreak

Following a terrible earthquake in 2010, the country of Haiti experienced an outbreak of cholera.[3] Cholera causes potentially fatal diarrhea and is usually prevented by maintaining clean water supplies. To prevent the further spread of the disease, United Nations officials not only supplied clean water, but also purchased supplies of a cholera vaccine.

Suppose we are charged with providing cholera vaccines for a village of 1,000 people. Based on data from prior outbreaks, we know that each person in Haiti who becomes infected with cholera typically infects three other people with the disease before recovering or dying from the illness, causing the outbreak to continue spreading. What is the minimum number of vaccines that should be purchased to stop the disease from continuing to spread in the village? Note that because of the biological concept of "herd immunity," which refers to the ability of a group of unvaccinated people to be protected from infection because they are surrounded by vaccinated people, we don't need to buy 1,000 vaccines. The extra money saved from vaccine purchases can be directed to other important public health activities, such as maintaining clean water supplies, so we wish to calculate the minimum number of vaccines necessary to stop the outbreak to optimize use of our precious resources.

Solution to Example Problem 3

This problem utilizes principles from the field of infectious disease epidemiology to study how to allocate limited resources. The question appeals to a fundamental epidemiological concept known as the "reproductive number," which is the number of times that a disease (in this case, cholera) reproduces itself among human hosts before the initial host dies or recovers. In our example, the local conditions in Haiti enabled the disease to reproduce itself in three people before the initial infected person died or recovered. Figure I.3 illustrates how we might visualize the chain of infection from a single person to the people whom they subsequently infect.

Our goal in this problem is to convert a chain of transmission from one that enables perpetual transmission, such as shown in Figure I.3, to a scenario in which sufficient people are vaccinated so that the chain of transmission cannot continue.

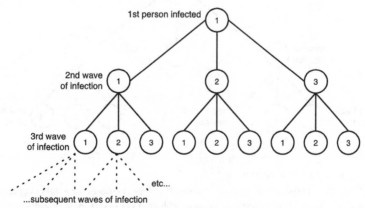

FIGURE I.3 **Example problem 3: The transmission of cholera. Every infected person produces three secondary infected people.**

Figure I.4 illustrates how a chain of transmission can be interrupted when people are vaccinated; but, as shown in the figure, if only a few people are vaccinated, the chain of transmission can continue. Our task is to determine what fraction of people must be vaccinated for the chain to eventually die out.

To solve this problem, we can derive an equation describing how vaccination affects the chain of transmission. If no people are vaccinated (Figure I.3), then with every next wave of infection, the number of people who are newly infected with cholera are the number who were previously infected multiplied by three. If one person is currently infected, then in the next wave of infection, three people will be infected; in the next wave of infection, nine people will be infected; and so on.

However, if people are vaccinated, then with every next wave of infection, the number of people who are newly infected with cholera are the number who were previously infected, times three, times the fraction of people who are unvaccinated (the fraction who remain susceptible to the disease). If one person is currently infected and one-third of people are vaccinated against the disease, then in the next wave of infection only two people will be infected instead of three; in the next wave of infection, only four people will be infected instead of nine (Figure I.4), and so on. That is, if f is the fraction of people who have been vaccinated in the village, then:

$$new\,infections = \left(old\,infections\right) \times 3 \times \left(1 - f\right). \qquad \text{[Equation I.5]}$$

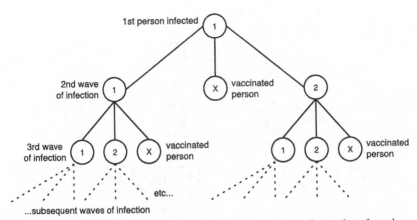

FIGURE I.4 Example problem 3 after vaccination. Vaccination reduces the number of people susceptible to infection. Shown here is an example with one out of every three villagers vaccinated. As shown, the number of secondary cases is reduced as vaccinated people interrupt the chain of transmission.

To stop an epidemic, we need the number of new people infected in the next wave of disease to be less than the number of people previously infected so that each next wave of disease has fewer and fewer people infected and the epidemic "dies out." Put another way:

$$\frac{new\,infections}{old\,infections} < 1. \qquad \text{[Equation I.6]}$$

The number of new infections divided by the number of old infections must be less than 1, meaning that fewer infections must occur with each subsequent wave of disease for the chain of transmission to eventually die out. We know from Equation I.5 that the number of new infections divided by the number of old infections is $3 \times (1 - f)$; hence, given Equations I.5 and I.6, we get:

$$3 \times (1 - f) < 1. \qquad \text{[Equation I.7]}$$

Solving for the value of f, we find that f must be greater than 0.666, or 66.6% of the population. In a village of 1,000 people, this means we must vaccinate at least 666 people to stop the outbreak.

In Chapter 10, we will formalize the equations we derived here and learn other fundamental equations that are commonly used to analyze infectious disease epidemics. We will apply these equations to more realistic circumstances, such as situations when the spread of disease occurs through complex social networks where some people are at much greater risk for infection than others.

Example Problem 4: Reducing Waiting Times for Drug Treatment

The City of San Francisco has established a centralized facility to help people addicted to drugs receive rehabilitation and treatment for addiction. People addicted to drugs who want to enter into a treatment program can sign up in a central office run by the City's health department. Because the number of available treatment spots (the supply) is less than the number of people signing up to receive treatment (the demand), there is a waiting list to receive treatment. Suppose that, on average, about 30 people sign up for treatment each month, and, on average, there are 10 openings for treatment spots each month. People are taken off the waiting list in the order they sign up, to be fair.

The City's health department Commissioner is interested in finding out how long people are able to wait in line before they relapse to drug use. He notices that the line is always around 100 people long, meaning that of the 30 people who sign up each month, 10 get treatment each month. The other 20 people—who were either already on the waiting list because they signed up a month or more earlier or just signed up this month—drop out of line, and the line stays about 100 people long. (This is a situation known as a "steady state" scenario, in which the waiting line is always around the same average length, a phenomenon we'll explore more in Chapter 5). Based on this information, how long can people wait in line until they relapse to drug use?

Solution to Example Problem 4

This is an example of a "queuing," or waiting time, problem. We can visualize the problem the way we visualize water flowing through pipes (Figure I.5): water comes into a bathtub (the waiting line), and water flows out through one of two drains (either the person gets treatment or the person falls out of line because she has relapsed to drug abuse).

We know that the rate at which people "flow" into the waiting line is 30 people per month, that the rate at which they "flow" out of line by getting into treatment is 10 people per month, and that the number of people waiting in line is around 100 people at any given time. We are solving for the average time that a person can wait in line before relapsing to drug use.

On average, 30 people enter the line each month, and hence 30 people must leave the line each month for the length of the line to be a stable number of 100 people. We know that 10 of those 30 people leaving the line are getting into a treatment slot, hence the other 20 must be dropping out by relapsing to drug use.

$$30\, people\, enter = 10\, people\, get\, in + 20\, people\, relapse.$$ [Equation I.8]

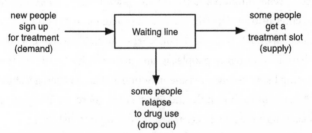

FIGURE I.5 Example problem 4: Modeling a waiting line for drug addiction treatment. As people sign up for drug addiction treatment, they wait in line and either receive treatment as treatment slots become available (right-hand side), or unfortunately relapse to drug use while waiting (bottom arrow).

Suppose the rate that people relapse to drug use is the letter d. The number of people relapsing is the number of people in line (100), times the rate at which they relapse. The rate at which they relapse is the inverse of the time they spend in line before they relapse (i.e., if I can wait in line for an average of 4 months before relapsing, then 1/(4 months), or I.25 per month, is my average probability of relapse per month or is the "rate" of relapse). To understand this concept of a "rate" more easily, suppose my chances of relapse are I.25 per month: then it would take 4 months before I have a probability of 1, or 100%, of having relapsed. Hence, the total number of people relapsing every month is 100 people times the dropout rate d per month, or $100d$ people per month dropping out of line by relapsing to drug use.

$$20\, people\, relapsing = 100 \times d\, people\, relapsing. \qquad \text{[Equation I.9]}$$

Solving for d, we find that the typical rate of relapse is 20/100 or 0.2/month, which means that the length of time people can wait in line before relapsing is 1/(0.2/month) = 5 months. In Chapter 5, we will solve queuing problems to identify answers to important healthcare system questions such as: if I increased the budget to provide 11 treatment slots instead of 10 per month, how many fewer people would relapse to drug use and instead get into treatment? How much would this cost, and would it be a cost-effective use of funds? And, more realistically, what happens if we're not at a "steady state," but the system is in flux?

Hopefully, the solutions to these four practice problems were not intuitive to readers and are sufficiently intriguing or even puzzling so that they leave many open questions among students reading the solutions. The student who finds these problems easy to solve is not an appropriate student for this book; it is the befuddled reader who wants more explanation, more scenarios to explore, and more opportunity to ask questions or present alternative approaches that we hope will be motivated by these problems. The rest of this book will offer the opportunity to pursue various questions about how to analyze different problems of these types, as well as a diverse array of other problems that arise in public health and healthcare systems. We will have the opportunity to explore various strategies to conceptualize common problems and derive solutions that are increasingly true to life's complexities. Despite the fact that these example problems are simplified scenarios, they illustrate an important principle for modeling: to start with a very basic problem and derive its solution first (as in the "steady state" case for example problem 4), just as Steinmetz started with a basic diagram of Ford's generator to piece together a solution. Ford's engineers were stymied by trying to desperately start with a complex solution to a complex problem, which can quickly become overwhelming. The principle of starting with the fundamentals of a problem and building up to a solution is an important strategy and an acquired skill we hope to confer through this text. Only after we master the simplest scenarios can we start to approach more complex situations that we often face in practice.

HOW TO USE THIS BOOK

This text is organized into three major sections and their associated chapters. The sections and even individual chapters may be read in isolation but have been intentionally organized to flow naturally from one another and provide a comprehensive overview of the current state of essential knowledge and the common tools employed by experts in modeling public health and healthcare systems. Hence, we would suggest that students and their instructors maintain the order of operations in the book.

The book's three parts include (1) foundations for modeling public health and healthcare systems, which includes key concepts, associated terminology, and fundamental equations for understanding models of disease screening and detection, decision making in public health and healthcare systems, and allocating scarce resources; (2) operations research techniques including ways to evaluate programs in community-based settings, optimally improve programs to ensure sufficient supply to meet demand, and evaluate problems involving complex schedules, teams, or tasks; and (3) simulation techniques that involve modern modeling strategies with computer modeling, including classical Markov and compartmental models, as well as newer microsimulation and agent-based simulation techniques.

Throughout each chapter, key concepts and modeling techniques are taught through a case-based approach in which problems are drawn from real-world settings, then solved in a manner that can derive a generalizable equation, method, or principle for broader application. The real-world problems are taken from healthcare organizations (e.g., the Kaiser Permanente healthcare system), nongovernmental organizations (e.g., Doctors Without Borders), public health departments (e.g., Los Angeles County Department of Public Health), and international agencies (e.g., World Health Organization) to motivate each section of each chapter. Each chapter uses a discovery-based learning approach in which one to three problems are solved to provide demonstration and derivation of a key method, followed by application of the method to solidify key concepts.

To ensure that the key concepts and methods are understood and solidified, each chapter is accompanied by either spreadsheets or code that can be run in the free statistical program R, which we discuss further later. These auxiliary materials are posted online at a permanent repository accessible at the URL: https://github.com/sanjaybasu/modelinghealthsystems.

SUPPLEMENTAL ONLINE MATERIAL

All models in the book are accompanied by code that is available online and can be run using the free program R, ensuring readers can replicate and extend the book's learning to their own research and work. The code is available at: https://github.com/sanjaybasu/modelinghealthsystems.

HOW TO BE PREPARED FOR THIS BOOK

This book is intended to be used by advanced undergraduate students (typically in their junior or senior years of college) and students enrolled in master's degree programs in public health, epidemiology, healthcare administration, health policy, or related fields. The mathematics background necessary for this course is limited to knowledge of basic calculus, including ordinary differential equations. For example, if we write the following differential equation:

$$\frac{\partial X(t)}{\partial t} = cX(t),$$

[Equation I.10]

readers should be able to interpret the equation as indicating that the rate of change in variable X for a change in variable t is a function of the constant c times the value of X at time t. In all cases, we have strived to ensure that any equations used throughout the text are explained thoroughly, with examples to maximize interpretability. In addition to having knowledge of basic calculus, readers should have taken an introductory-level course in probability and statistics, which would cover topics such as probability distributions (e.g., what is a Gaussian or normal, versus a skewed, distribution), the Central Limit Theorem, and basic principles of statistical sampling and regression.

In addition to a basic background in probability and calculus, readers should be prepared to use both of the two software packages employed in this course: (1) Microsoft Excel (or an equivalent spreadsheet program with a Solver function, such as the freely downloadable software LibreOffice) and (2) the free statistical program R, which can be downloaded from https://www.r-project.org/. Those students who have not previously used R are recommended to take the free introduction to R available at http://tryr.codeschool.com/, although this book will include a detailed introduction to the program.

We stress that we do not expect students using this book to have any prior experience in computer programming. We will introduce the preceding tools when they are needed in the course, and, at this point, students should simply download these programs to have them available when they are introduced in later chapters of this book.

PART ONE
Foundations

1

FUNDAMENTALS

In this chapter, we define and provide examples of several key terms used in public health and healthcare modeling research. We begin by clarifying the differences between key terms used to describe rates of disease (incidence, prevalence, and mortality) as well as the performance characteristics of tests used to detect disease (sensitivity, specificity, positive predictive value, and negative predictive value), prevent or treat disease (odds ratios, relative risks), understand studies (case-control, cohort, and randomized controlled trials), and avoid common study problems (bias, confounding).

INCIDENCE, PREVALENCE AND MORTALITY: AN EXAMPLE FROM HIV IN UGANDA

In the 1990s, human immunodeficiency virus (HIV) ravaged entire countries and debate ensued regarding the most appropriate strategy to reduce transmission of the disease. Public health experts advocated for wider distribution of condoms to prevent sexual transmission of HIV, but officials at the US White House (under then-President George W. Bush) argued that such an approach would legitimize unsafe sex. Instead, White House officials declared that "abstinence-only" educational programs were effective for preventing HIV infections. They reported that, when broadly instituted, abstinence-only programs were shown to generate substantial reductions in the number of people with HIV over time.

Public health experts were skeptical, but they did not find any problems with the data collection that led to the reports released by the White House. The number of HIV-positive individuals had been studied appropriately by surveilling a similar population of people over many years in areas without major migration and in locations where other factors contributing to HIV transmission (the local economy, for example) had not changed over the study period. If the data were in fact correct, what reason—other than the success of abstinence-only programs—might explain why the number of people infected with HIV had declined after the introduction of the programs in Uganda?

To answer this question, we need to clarify three key terms used to describe rates of disease: incidence, prevalence, and mortality. Perhaps the most straightforward way to remember the important distinction between these terms is to visualize a bathtub, as shown in Figure 1.1.

If the bathtub reflects the state of HIV in an area, then we can conceptualize the *flow* of water into the bathtub as the *incidence* rate of HIV, or the number of people over a period of time (per week, per month, or per year, to give a few examples) who are newly infected with HIV in the studied Ugandan communities.

We can conceptualize the *level* of water in the bathtub as the *prevalence* of disease, or the number of people at a particular time of a study who are infected with HIV. Unlike a rate of incidence, the prevalence of a disease reflects a single point in time—not a change in people over a period of time. The statistics used by the White House were prevalence statistics. In other words, White House officials compared the number of people with HIV in the years prior to the abstinence-only education program to the number of people with HIV in the years after the abstinence-only education program.

Finally, we can conceptualize the *flow* of water out of the bathtub as the *mortality* rate from HIV, or the number of people over a period of time who have died from HIV or HIV-related complications.

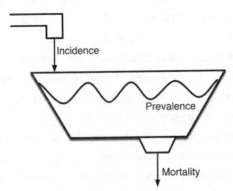

FIGURE 1.1 The bathtub analogy for deciphering incidence, prevalence, and mortality. We can conceptualize the *flow* of water into the bathtub as the *incidence* rate, or the number of people over a period of time (per week, per month, or per year, to give a few examples) who newly acquire the disease. We can conceptualize the *level* of water in the bathtub at the *prevalence* of disease, or the number of people at a particular time of a study who have the disease. Unlike a rate of incidence, the prevalence of a disease reflects a single point in time—not a change in people overF a period of time. We can conceptualize the *flow* of water out of the bathtub as the *mortality* rate from the disease, or the number of people over a period of time who have died from the disease.

As illustrated by the bathtub analogy, incidence and mortality are *rates* of disease—they indicate the number of newly infected or dead persons per unit time. In contrast, prevalence is a *level* of disease (the number of people with the disease at the moment of measurement). Using these definitions, can you determine how White House officials may have incorrectly ascertained the effectiveness of abstinence-only programming?

There are two reasons why the level of water in a bathtub might decrease. First, the faucet could be turned down, causing less water to enter the bathtub through the faucet than leaves the bathtub through the drain per unit time. Alternatively, water could exit the bathtub more rapidly (suppose a plug is removed from the drain, for example) such that more water leaves the bathtub through the drain than enters the bathtub through the faucet per unit time.

Similarly, the prevalence of a disease might decline for one of two reasons: either fewer people are getting the disease than are dying from the disease (the incidence rate has declined relative to the mortality rate), or more people are dying from the disease than are getting the disease (the mortality rate has increased relative to the incidence rate).

Unfortunately, in the case of HIV in Uganda, the incidence rate of HIV had not declined as a consequence of effective abstinence-only programs. Instead, scarce opportunities for treatment caused the mortality rate to continue increasing in the population. Hence, the diminishing prevalence of HIV-positive individuals in Uganda during this time did not reflect the effectiveness of abstinence-only programming, but the rapid and deadly decline faced by patients who contracted HIV.[1]

OPTIMIZATION: A STARTING MODEL FOR RESOURCE ALLOCATION

In 2013, a large outbreak of *Salmonella* caused several people across the United States to fall ill. Outbreaks of *Salmonella* are typically caused by contaminated chicken or eggs and are frequently traced back to a single producer that mishandled and contaminated food items. The outbreak in 2013, however, caused people to fall ill from *Salmonella* infections in regions across many distant states, suggesting that a single grocery store was not to blame. Officials at the US Centers for Disease Control and Prevention (CDC) visited the grocery stores where those affected had purchased chicken or eggs. They discovered that a common brand of chicken had been purchased by all of the infected individuals and traced that brand to a single factory that had mishandled and contaminated a large batch of chicken with bird feces. This contaminated chicken was packaged and subsequently distributed to grocery stores across the country.

In the investigation that followed, the CDC learned that the factory liable for the contamination event was not under an active inspection program. Usually, the active inspection program sent inspectors to factories where they could identify contamination events, discard contaminated food items, and consequently prevent disease outbreaks. The revelation that an inspector had not been present at the implicated factory caused an uproar among consumer advocacy groups, who then called their Congressional representatives to complain. The Congressional representatives, in turn, called the US Department of Agriculture (USDA) to demand an explanation. USDA officials argued that they had a limited budget to pay for inspectors. More specifically, out of every 100 factories that handled food products, the USDA had only the budget to provide inspectors at about 10 factories.

To minimize the chances of missing a contamination event, the USDA classified factories as "high risk" or "normal risk" based on whether they processed foods that required careful handling (such as meat products) or foods that were not particularly dangerous. Suppose that out of every 100 factories, 20 of them were classified as high-risk and the other 80 were classified as normal risk (Figure 1.2). How could we, if we were USDA administrators, minimize the chances of missing a contamination event by distributing our 10 inspectors among the 100 factories?

To answer this question, we can define a few terms to make the problem easier. Suppose we call the variable f the *search capacity*, which we define as *the fraction of our inspectors whom we devote to high-risk factories*. For example, if $f = 0.2$, then 20% of our inspectors will be directed to high-risk factories. Therefore, $1 - f$ must represent the fraction of our inspectors devoted to normal-risk factories (0.8, or 80%, in this example). We can also specify that the goal of our work is to maximize the *capture probability* of finding a contaminated batch of food, which is *the probability*

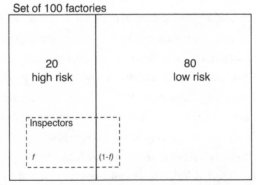

FIGURE 1.2 Optimization problem of distributing inspectors among factories. Suppose that out of every 100 factories, 20 of them were classified as high-risk and the other 80 were classified as normal risk. We call the variable f the *search capacity*, which we define as the fraction of our inspectors who we devote to high-risk factories.

that if a contamination event has already occurred, our inspector will find it. We can assume, for simplicity, that our inspectors are highly observant and detect every contamination event at the factory to which they are assigned. Hence, the capture probability is the probability that if a contamination event has occurred, it has occurred in a factory to which we have assigned an inspector.

This dilemma is an example of an *optimization problem*—a situation in which we wish to maximize or minimize something (in this case, maximizing our capture probability) by choosing a course of action that is subject to certain constraints. In this case, for instance, we have to determine how to best allocate a limited number of inspectors among a larger set of factories.

We can solve our problem—how to distribute our inspectors to maximize our chances of finding a contamination event—by calculating our probability of finding a contamination event if it has happened in a high-risk factory. First, suppose we choose to devote all of our resources to high-risk factories, meaning we allocate all 10 of our inspectors to high-risk factories. What is our probability of finding a contamination event if it has happened in a high-risk factory? Given our resources, we can screen only 10 of the total 100 factories. Since 20 factories are high-risk, we can detect, at most, contamination events at 10/20, or 50%, of high-risk factories.

Suppose, however, that we set $f = 0.7$. That is, we assign 70% of our inspectors to high-risk factories. Under this new allocation of resources, the proportion of high-risk factories to be inspected will be:

$$0.7 * 10 / 20 = 0.35, \hspace{4cm} \text{[Equation 1.1]}$$

or 35%. Hence, there is a 35% chance of detecting a contamination event that happens in a high-risk factory if we set $f = 0.7$.

Similarly, what is our probability of finding a contamination event if it has happened in a normal-risk factory? By analogous reasoning, we have devoted $1 - f = 0.3$ (or 30%) of our inspectors to normal-risk factories. Since there are 80 normal-risk factories, if we begin with the scenario in which we devote all of our inspectors to normal-risk factories, we can inspect at most 10 of the 80 factories. However, we have devoted only 30% of our inspectors to normal-risk factories, so the probability that we detect a contamination event that happens in a normal-risk factory is:

$$0.3 * 10 / 80 = 0.0375, \hspace{4cm} \text{[Equation 1.2]}$$

or 3.75%. This is a remarkably depressing outcome. If a lay-person read a newspaper that said, "We devoted most of our inspectors, 70% of them, to inspecting high-risk factories, and devoted 30% to normal-risk factories to prevent contamination from slipping between the cracks," they may be satisfied with this allocation of resources. However, our limited capacity permits us to inspect only 10% of factories, so even devoting 70% of resources to the high-risk group leaves only a 35% chance—less than a flip of a coin—of catching a contamination event if it occurs at a high-risk factory. Similarly, this allocation of resources means we have a 3.75% chance of catching a contamination event if it has occurred at a low-risk factory. In short, our resource constraints dramatically compromise our chances of identifying a contamination event at low- and high-risk factors.

Nevertheless, we can take the same action typically taken by the USDA and public health departments across the country to maximize the impact of the inspectors we have available to us. Large agencies or departments commonly use historical data to identify a strategy that maximizes their capture probability. Suppose, for example, that we have historical information indicating the frequency with which contamination events have previously occurred at high-risk and low-risk factories. We can specify the quantity q as the fraction of the time that the contamination event occurred in a high-risk factory; therefore, $1 - q$ would correspond to the fraction of the time that the contamination event occurred in a normal-risk factory.

What would the capture probability be in terms of f and q?

We can define the capture probability as the sum of two quantities:

$$
\text{Capture probability} = \left[\begin{pmatrix} \text{probability of finding a contamination} \\ \text{event if that event has happened in} \\ \text{a high-risk factory} \end{pmatrix} \\ \times \begin{pmatrix} \text{probability that the contamination} \\ \text{event has happened in a high-risk factory} \end{pmatrix} \right] \\ + \left[\begin{pmatrix} \text{probability of finding a contamination event if} \\ \text{that event has happened in a normal-risk factory} \end{pmatrix} \\ \times \begin{pmatrix} \text{probability that the contamination has happened} \\ \text{in a normal-risk factory} \end{pmatrix} \right]
$$

[Equation 1.3]

We can define each of these component entities in terms of f and q:

The probability of finding a contamination event if it happens in a high-risk factory is $f * 10/20$.

The probability of contamination in a high-risk factory is q.

The probability of finding a contamination event if it happens in a normal-risk factory is $(1 - f) * 10/80$.

The probability of contamination in a normal-risk factory is $(1 - q)$.

Therefore, the capture probability, $P(capture)$, is:

$$P(capture) = \frac{f \times 10}{20} \times q + \frac{(1-f) \times 10}{80} \times (1-q).$$ [Equation 1.4]

This expression is not particularly simple to interpret, but suppose we rearrange the expression as follows to have the equation express the capture probability as a function of one number times f, plus another number:

$$
\begin{aligned}
P(capture) &= \frac{f \times 10}{20} \times q + \frac{(1-f) \times 10}{80} \times (1-q) \\
&= \frac{1}{2} fq + \frac{1}{8}(1-f)(1-q) \\
&= \frac{1}{2} fq + \frac{1}{8}(1-q) - \frac{1}{8}f(1-q) \\
&= \frac{1}{2} fq - \frac{1}{8}f(1-q) + \frac{1}{8}(1-q) \\
&= \left(\frac{1}{2}q - \frac{1}{8}(1-q)\right)f + \frac{1}{8}(1-q) \\
&= (slope) \times f + intercept.
\end{aligned}
$$ [Equation 1.5]

Here, we have derived a function that describes the capture probability in terms of some numerical quantity multiplied by the search capacity f, plus a constant number. Readers may recognize this function as a standard linear equation in which the first expression is a slope and the second expression is an intercept on the y-axis. In other words, the capture probability can be generally expressed in the form of a line with an intercept and a slope.

How does this help us? By deriving Equation 1.5, we have identified an expression that, when solved, allows us to maximize the capture probability for any situation in which we need to allocate resources. If our objective is to maximize our capture probability, for example, we can observe that the best value of f for maximizing the capture probability will depend on whether the slope of our expression is positive or negative. If the slope is positive, then increasing f will increase the capture probability. Thus, we can maximize our capture probability by making f as large as possible (by setting f to a value of 1). Conversely, if the slope in Equation 1.5 is negative, then the capture probability increases by decreasing f. Hence, if the slope is negative, we can maximize our capture probability by making f as small as possible (by setting it to a value of 0).

This reasoning grants us a solution to our optimization problem. To maximize the capture probability, we can set the value of f to 1 in cases when our slope is positive or set f equal to 0 in cases when our slope is negative. In our contamination example, deriving an equation with a positive slope would indicate that our capture probability is maximized when all of our inspectors are allocated to high-risk factories. In mathematical terms, this means that we should set the value of f to 1 if:

$$\left(\frac{1}{2}q - \frac{1}{8}(1-q)\right) > 0.$$ [Equation 1.6]

Simplifying to solve for q, we obtain:

$$\left(\frac{1}{2}q + \frac{1}{8}q - \frac{1}{8}\right) > 0$$
$$\frac{5}{8}q > \frac{1}{8}$$
$$q > \frac{1}{5}.$$ [Equation 1.7]

Hence, whenever our historical data tell us that more than 1/5 (or 20%) of contamination events have occurred in high-risk factories, we should set the value of f to 1 by placing all of our inspectors in high-risk factories. Conversely, if q is less than 20%, we should set the value of f to 0 by placing all of our inspectors in normal-risk factories. If q is exactly 20%, then from Equation 1.5 we see that the slope would be zero—no matter what value we choose for f, the capture probability will always equal the intercept $(1/8 * (1 - q))$.

In this example, we used historical data regarding previous contamination events to solve our optimization problem and determine how to maximize our capture probability. In the process, we derived a generalizable equation that may be applied for any problem in which we must allocate resources among distinct entities (inspectors allocated to factories, in our example). To derive our solution for other circumstances, we can retrace the three steps we took to arrive at our solution: (1) estimate the probability of detecting a problem (e.g., a contamination event at a food factory) based on the resources allocated to each entity (e.g., high-risk and normal-risk factories); (2) create an expression for the capture probability in terms of the probability of detecting a problem at each entity, multiplied by the historical rate of a problem occurring at each entity; and (3) identify under which conditions the expression for the capture probability will be maximized.

In working through this example, we created our first model—one that required us to define some new concepts, work systematically through a problem, and arrive at a generalizable solution. In more complex cases, we can expand our approach to allocate more than one resource to more than two entities. We can also generalize our approach to circumstances in which we need to allocate resources with more constraints—that is, situations where we need to consider multiple requirements as we choose how to distribute our resources. We will address such problems using computational tools in Chapter 3.

SENSITIVITY, SPECIFICITY, AND PREDICTIVE VALUES: AN EXAMPLE FROM LUPUS SCREENING

The model of allocation processes that we derived from our example of *Salmonella* contamination was based on a key assumption: when we allocate resources such as inspectors to a factory, our resources will be perfectly effective: every inspector will find every contamination event at his or her assigned factory.

Reality, of course, is far less than perfect.

When evaluating screening strategies, we must often decide between imperfect tools. For most medical and public health situations, we have to carefully quantify how far our tools are from perfection to ensure that we use our tests and tools as well as possible.

Suppose we take the example of screening patients for systematic lupus erythematosus (SLE), a rare disease affecting about 0.2% of the population and commonly known as "lupus." Lupus is an autoimmune disease, meaning it is triggered by self-reactive antibodies that attack a person's own organs, joints, and skin. Unfortunately, many people who have lupus are not diagnosed until their antibodies have already caused severe and irreversible damage. If caught in the earlier stages of disease, however, people with lupus can receive medical treatment that can prevent serious complications.

The Lupus Foundation of America started a campaign to encourage people with symptoms characteristic of lupus to contact their medical providers and request screening. Billboards and radio and television advertisements, as well as social media campaigns, were started to encourage young women to receive a screening test for lupus, known as the antinuclear antibody (ANA) test.

The Foundation argued that the ANA test would be an excellent recommendation for most people since it was known to have a high capture probability for detecting lupus. However, medical groups worried that recommending wide testing would cause a serious problem. To visualize the problem, we can visualize a scenario in which the ANA test is applied to a population of 10,000 people. Typically, such data are portrayed using a *contingency table* (Table 1.1) which summarizes not only the number of people who test positive or negative using the ANA test, but also the number of people who are later confirmed to truly have (or not have) lupus.

From this table, we can observe that the capture probability of detecting a patient with lupus, if they truly have lupus, is 100%.[2] Out of 20 people who had the disease, all 20 test positive. The capture probability *of detecting a person with the disease* is commonly referred to as a test's *sensitivity*. We can calculate the sensitivity as the

Table 1.1 Contingency table of the number of people who tested positive or negative using the ANA test and the number of people later confirmed to truly have (or not have) lupus

	Actually Have Disease (10,000 * 0.2% = 20)	Do Not Actually Have Disease (10,000 * 99.8% = 9,980)
Test positive	20	1,397
Test negative	0	8,583

number of people testing positive who actually have the disease, divided by the total number of people having the disease:

$$\text{Sensitivity} = (\text{true positives}) / (\text{all persons with the disease}). \qquad [\text{Equation 1.8}]$$

A problem with the ANA test, however, is that only 86% of people who did not have lupus ended up having a negative test (8,593/9,980). The probability of *correctly identifying a person who does not have the disease* is known as a test's *specificity*:

$$\text{Specificity} = (\text{true negatives}) / (\text{all persons without the disease}). \qquad [\text{Equation 1.9}]$$

The low specificity of the ANA test generated many "false-positive" results. In other words, 1,397 people who did not have lupus were incorrectly labeled as having lupus based on the ANA test.

We can fill out a more complete contingency table to help us determine the value of a particular medical test; in Table 1.2, we add key terms that are commonly used to label people who appear in each cell of the table and summarize the value of a test in terms of the *positive predictive value* (the probability of having the disease if a

Table 1.2 Complete contingency table to help determine the value of a particular medical test

	Actually Have Disease (20)	Do Not Actually Have Disease (9,980)	
Test positive	True positive (20)	False positive (1,397)	Positive predictive value = 20/(20 + 1,397) = 1%
Test negative	False negative (0)	True negative (8,583)	Negative predictive value = 8,583/(0 + 8,583) = 100%
	Sensitivity = 20/(20 + 0) = 100%	Specificity = 8,583/ (1,397 + 8,583) = 86%	

person tests positive) and *negative predictive value* (the probability of not having the disease if the person tests negative):

As shown in Table 1.2, the positive predictive value for the ANA test is very low, so having a positive test does not necessarily mean that a person has lupus. (In fact, patients with positive test results most likely do not have lupus.) Conversely, the negative predictive value for the ANA test is 100%, so if a person is negative, they can rest assured that they do not have the disease. Hence, the ANA test may still be useful, but only for ruling out the disease among people truly suspected of having the illness. For the general population of patients having aches and pains without any more specific symptoms or family history of lupus, the ANA test is more likely to produce a "false-positive" result and cause needless worry.

A common pair of acronyms used to remember when tests are useful is SPIN and SNOUT: a SPecific test helps us to rule IN the disease (diagnose someone), whereas a test with high SeNsitivity helps us to rule OUT the disease (if a person is negative, they can be reassured that they are unlikely to have it). Tests are rarely highly sensitive and highly specific, so we usually apply them in sequence: first, we use a test with high sensitivity to rule out many people who don't have the disease, then administer a test with high specificity among the persons who tested positive to diagnose people with the disease.

RISKS AND STUDY DESIGNS

Detecting disease accurately is critical to nearly every public health or healthcare task, but the natural next step is to provide an effective intervention that reduces the morbidity and mortality caused by that disease. For example, many programs in the United States seek to detect people with "pre-diabetes" (a state of not yet having irreversible diabetes but being at high risk for eventually developing the disease). Persons labeled as having pre-diabetes may benefit from an effective nutrition and physical activity program that delays or prevents the onset of full-blown diabetes. Similarly, people who have an early stage of disease may be able to receive effective pharmaceutical treatments to prevent complications or death from the disease. How can we know if an intervention is actually effective?

A similar problem arises if we wish to detect whether an environmental agent may be increasing the risk of disease—for example, whether exposure to a chemical might cause cancer or whether people with certain health-related behaviors (e.g., tobacco smoking) have a higher risk of lung disease.

Just as we created a contingency table to determine how many people with a disease had a positive or negative test result, we can create analogous contingency tables to determine if our interventions improve the chances of living a healthy life or whether environmental or personal characteristics worsen the chances of living a healthy life. In Table 1.3, we illustrate such a contingency table:

Table 1.3 Contingency table illustrating the relationship between exposure to a chemical and cancer incidence

	Got Cancer	Didn't Get Cancer
Exposed to chemical	15	70
Not exposed to chemical	5	150

In Table 1.3, the rows refer to whether or not a person was exposed to a chemical, and the columns tell us whether or not these people later got cancer or remained cancer-free. Typically, these data are obtained from a *cohort study* (also commonly called a longitudinal cohort study), in which we follow a group of people over time and evaluate how many of the people exposed to a chemical developed cancer and how many people not exposed to the chemical got cancer.

As shown in Table 1.3, the absolute number of people who didn't get cancer is, thankfully, higher than those who did. Also, as expected, fewer people were exposed to the chemical than were unexposed. How do we quantify the extent to which the chemical exposure is associated with cancer?

Epidemiologists typically quantify the risk of disease given an exposure as a *relative risk (RR)*, sometimes also referred to as a "risk ratio," which is calculated as:

$$RR = \frac{(Exposed\ and\ got\ cancer)/(Total\ exposed)}{(Not\ exposed\ and\ got\ cancer)/(Total\ not\ exposed)}. \qquad \text{[Equation 1.10]}$$

In the case of the example shown in Table 1.3, the relative risk would be [15/(15 + 70)]/[5/(5 + 150)] = 5.5, which can be interpreted as suggesting that there is more than a fivefold higher risk of getting cancer if a person was exposed to the chemical than if they were not exposed.

In the case of some rare diseases, it is hard to perform a cohort study because even people who are exposed very rarely get the disease, and only extremely large sample sizes (read: very expensive studies) would be able to capture enough people who eventually develop the rare disease to calculate a relative risk. In this circumstance, epidemiologists typically perform a *case-control study* (also commonly called a retrospective case-control study), which involves finding people who already have the disease and asking them whether they were previously exposed to the chemical or factor under study. These *cases* are compared to people who don't have the disease (*controls*). The problem with case-control studies is that they only sample groups of people with and without the disease instead of the entire population. Thus, we are unsure how many people in the overall population were actually exposed to the chemical and how many were not. This complicates our ability to determine an accurate denominator in our risk estimates. In case-control studies, epidemiologists will calculate an *odds ratio (OR)* instead of calculating a relative risk:

$$OR = \frac{\left(Exposed\,and\,got\,cancer\right) / \left(Exposed\,and\,didn't\,get\,cancer\right)}{\left(Not\,exposed\,and\,got\,cancer\right) / \left(Not\,exposed\,and\,didn't\,get\,cancer\right)}.$$

[Equation 1.11]

If Table 1.3 were data from a case-control study, then the OR would be (15/70)/(5/150) = 6.4. Here, we interpret the odds ratio by saying that the "odds" of getting cancer when exposed to the chemical are more than sixfold the "odds" of getting cancer if a person is not exposed to the chemical. The term "odds" is deceptive, however, because it is a ratio of two factors in the contingency table, not a probability. For very rare diseases, the odds ratio and the relative risk will be similar values because the number of people who are exposed and didn't get the disease and the number of people not exposed who didn't get the disease are relatively large; hence, these values are similar to the total number of people exposed and the total number who did not get the disease, making Equation 1.11 very similar to Equation 1.10.

If we wish to determine if an exposure results in disease, then cohort and case-control studies are reasonable investigative strategies, especially because it is usually unethical or impractical to subject people to an exposure to determine if they eventually get the disease under study. Conversely, if we wish to determine if an intervention (such as vaccine or pharmaceutical) can help prevent or treat a disease, it is often ethical and practical to subject people to the intervention to determine if it truly mitigates disease risk or disease mortality. The beneficial effects of interventions are often best tested using a *randomized controlled trial* (RCT). An RCT involves randomly flipping a coin and assigning some people to get the intervention (e.g., a new pharmaceutical medication) and assigning other people to a "placebo" group (e.g., an empty pill capsule). The benefit of an RCT is that, in the process of randomly assigning people to the intervention group or comparison group, *confounding factors*—that is, factors correlated with both the intervention and the outcome of interest—are distributed equally into both groups. If confounders are distributed equally between groups, they are washed out from the statistical analysis of the intervention, thus allowing us to correctly estimate the impact of the intervention on the disease risk or mortality.

For example, suppose that we want to know if a particular vitamin was associated with a lower risk of heart disease. If we just did a cohort study of how many people were exposed to the vitamin and how many got heart disease, we might find data such as those shown in Table 1.4:

Table 1.4 Contingency table illustrating the relationship between heart disease and vitamin intake

	Got Heart Disease	Didn't Get Heart Disease
Ate vitamin	3	80
Didn't eat vitamin	7	60

Based on the data from Table 1.4, we might conclude that the vitamin is very effective at preventing heart disease because the relative risk is RR = [3/(3 + 80)]/ [7/(7 + 60)] = 0.3, meaning that people who took the vitamin only got heart disease about one-third as much as people not taking the vitamin. However, a confounding factor may account for these results. Suppose that the vitamin in question is found disproportionately in green vegetables. Perhaps the vitamin leads to lower incidence of heart disease, or perhaps something else in green vegetables is responsible for the lower incidence of heart disease (fiber, for example). Other factors like fiber may "travel alongside" the vitamin and generate the reduction in heart disease, but we have wrongly attributed the benefit to the vitamin instead of to fiber.

An RCT would be able to separate out the impact of the vitamin from the impact of "fellow travelers" (confounders) to determine whether the vitamin is actually producing the benefits observed. An RCT could, for example, be designed so that some people were randomly given a pill containing only the vitamin and other people were randomly given a pill that was just an empty capsule (a placebo). Because we randomly assigned people to the vitamin or placebo pill, the number of people in each group who eat green vegetables should be roughly equal if we have a large-enough sample size—consequently washing out the effect of green vegetables because both groups would have people with high and low green vegetable consumption and the only effect left would be from the vitamin itself. We could then recalculate the relative risk from the RCT data knowing that the outcome should be just the effect of the intervention (the vitamin) rather than confounding factors (like fiber).

RCTs are not always possible, as in cases when it would be unethical to randomize people to harmful exposures. Unfortunately, medical history does have examples of highly unethical studies, including the infamous Tuskegee Syphilis Study in which Black men in the southern United States were intentionally prevented from receiving treatment for syphilis to understand how the disease affected their bodies. Hence, it is important for us to continue doing case-control and cohort studies to identify how natural occurrences might affect disease risk.

Relative risks and odds ratios will be frequently incorporated into our models, particularly when we seek to simulate the benefit incurred from an intervention or assess how rates of disease may be affected if exposure to environmental or behavioral factors were to change.

BIAS

When we gather data to put into our models, we usually have to think about whether those data are *biased*, or producing a false estimate of reality.

Two forms of bias are particularly important for modelers of public health and healthcare systems to be aware of. The first—*selection bias*—refers to the problem of "comparing apples to oranges," or having one group of people compared to a group of people who are very different from them. For example, a famous study reported that workers in shipyards who had been exposed to radiation many years ago were actually healthier and had lower rates of death than people who did not get exposed to radiation.[3] At face value, the study seems likely to be wrong—but why? Further investigation revealed that the people who conducted the study had compared workers in the shipyard to a broad population of people. Importantly, workers in the shipyard were only selected from a relatively healthy population of young men who had passed an initial physical exam. By contrast, the shipyard workers were compared to a broad population including very elderly people. Hence, the study was biased, and a proper comparison would have been between young healthy men who entered the shipyards and young healthy men who did not.

Another example of selection bias was observed in recent studies of nutrition. A study compared obesity rates among people who received "food stamps," a form of financial assistance for low-income populations in need of food. A study compared the food stamp recipients to nonrecipients and found that persons using food stamps had higher rates of obesity. The authors concluded that food stamps themselves led to obesity. However, the people receiving food stamps tended to live in neighborhoods that had higher concentrations of fast food restaurants and fewer grocers selling fresh fruits and vegetables. Hence, selection bias could have occurred, and a fairer comparison would have been between food stamp recipients and nonrecipients in similar neighborhoods.[4,5]

A second form of bias is known as *information or observation bias*, sometimes also called misclassification bias. Information or observational bias refers to a problem that arises when an exposure or outcome is measured incorrectly. This type of measurement error can affect both groups equally. For example, suppose a laboratory test is used to assess a person's cholesterol levels to see if cholesterol relates to heart disease. If the laboratory test underestimates everyone's cholesterol values by the same amount, it can produce *nondifferential misclassification*—meaning that people with both high and low cholesterol values are equally affected. This is nevertheless a problem because we will not know the true association between correctly measured cholesterol levels and heart disease.

Differential misclassification—when measurement error is greater among one group than another—poses an even greater problem. A classical example of differential misclassification is when people who are affected by some exposure tend to remember having a problem more than people who were not exposed. In a study of the chemical Agent Orange (a substance used by the US military in the Vietnam War), for example, pilots in the US Air Force who had been exposed to the chemical remembered having skin rashes after exposure much more than pilots who hadn't been exposed, but objective physical exam records show that the two groups of pilots actually had the same rate of skin rashes. Pilots exposed to Agent Orange were more attuned to their rashes (they remembered them more readily) than those who were not exposed.[6] Another example of information bias occurs with mothers who have children with congenital birth defects. Mothers whose children are born with birth defects recall being exposed to medications more than mothers whose children are born without defects, even if they took the same number of medications.[7]

2

VALUE

In this chapter, we seek to answer the question: how much should we pay for a public health program? We often have to decide how to allocate funds to different public health programs or decide whether a new medical test or treatment is worth the cost. How can we make such decisions fairly? We'll first work through some examples of *decision trees* that are commonly used to make these judgments in a rigorous and fair way. We'll create some decision trees to solve *value of information* problems, which are used to perform *cost-benefit analysis* to determine whether we want to pay for a new service, test, or treatment if we are focused on lowering the costs of our operations. We'll then understand how to perform *cost-effectiveness analysis* to identify under what circumstances a more expensive new service, test, or treatment might be worth the cost because it meaningfully improves health outcomes.

DECISION TREES

We often have to make complex decisions about what course of action to pursue; in public health and healthcare service delivery, those decisions can have life-or-death consequences. To make the best decisions based on the information we have available, we often construct decision trees: graphical representations of a decision and its potential consequences. Decision trees represent one of the most fundamental strategies for modeling public health and healthcare problems and serve as a foundation for the future models that we will develop to analyze complex decisions.

To understand how to build and solve a decision tree, suppose we have a common decision problem: whether to administer a new experimental drug to a patient. Suppose a new experimental drug has been designed to treat a deadly form of kidney cancer. If a person undergoes treatment for the cancer with a standard existing drug, they have a 15% chance of survival and an 85% chance of death. With the new experimental drug, they have a 40% chance of remission and a 60% chance of death. However, among those people who experienced a remission, 50% survived and 50% later died.

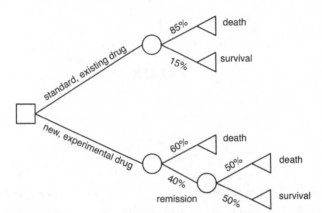

FIGURE 2.1 A decision tree for whether to recommend the new, experimental drug to a patient with kidney cancer, which specifies the probability of each outcome. If a person undergoes treatment for the cancer with a standard, existing drug, they have a 15% chance of survival and an 85% chance of death. With the new, experimental drug, they have a 40% chance of remission and a 60% chance of death. However, among those people who experienced a remission, 50% survived and 50% later died. We typically designate the start of a decision tree with a square, and each "chance node" or decision branching point with a circle. Triangles then designate the endpoint (sometimes called a leaf node or terminal node) of each branch. Next to each decision branch is the probability of traveling along that branch. Next to each node is the value of the node.

If we wish to determine whether to recommend the new experimental drug to a patient with kidney cancer, how might we rationally compare the standard existing drug to the new experimental drug?

To solve this problem, we can draw all possible outcomes on a decision tree which specifies both the probability of each outcome and the "value" of each outcome (see Figure 2.1). For this problem, we value the outcome of survival, so we will specify that an outcome has value 0 if a person dies and value 1 if a person survives; this designation will allow us to easily calculate and compare the probability of survival between the two groups.

As shown in Figure 2.1, we typically designate the start of a decision tree with a square and each "chance node" or decision branching point with a circle. Triangles then designate the endpoint (sometimes called a leaf node or terminal node) of each branch. Next to each decision branch is the probability of traveling along that branch. Next to each node is the value of the node.

To "solve" the decision tree, we start from the right-hand side of the tree and calculate the probability of survival for each node, "rolling back" ultimately to the first node (the root node) to determine the ultimate expected probability of survival for our patient if they were offered one therapy or another.

For example, suppose we start with the top node corresponding to the standard existing drug. We see there is an 85% probability of death and a 15% probability of survival, leading to a "value" (probability of survival) of $0.85 \times 0 + 0.15 \times 1 = 0.15$.

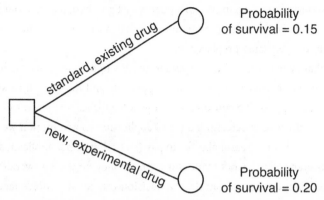

FIGURE 2.2 Solution to the decision tree for whether to recommend the new, experimental drug to a patient with kidney cancer

Similarly, if we start with the bottom-right node we can see that, with remission, there is a probability of survival of 0.5. Because there is a 60% probability of death and a 40% probability of remission with the new experimental drug, we can calculate that the overall probability of survival with the new experimental drug is $0.6 \times 0 + 0.4 \times 0.5 \times 1 = 0.20$ (the 0.4×0.5 is the probability of remission multiplied by the probability of survival given remission), as shown in Figure 2.2.

The "solved" decision tree makes our decision fairly clear: we should recommend the new experimental drug to our patient, assuming that survival is the primary outcome we are basing our decision on.

THE VALUE OF INFORMATION

Solving a decision tree is a nice way to organize our thinking, but often the information we have available is not as certain as in the case of comparing one drug to another. For many decisions we make in public health and healthcare, we have to determine whether it's better to make a decision based on the current information we have or spend time and resources trying to find out more information to make an even better decision. Every time we spend time or resources, we lose the opportunity to do other things.

Here is a classic example: back in the early 2000s, the US Department of Veteran's Affairs (VA) was running out of pharmacists to staff several of its hospitals, which serve veterans returning from war with serious injuries. The VA decided to undertake a major hiring blitz by offering an up-front bonus of $50,000 for every pharmacist who was hired. Unfortunately, some of the pharmacists who were hired turned out to have poor performance reports and had to be fired. Suppose that about 20% had to be fired and the other 80% were fine. The process of hiring a new pharmacist then had to start all over again. When a pharmacist got fired, it cost about $1,000 to do the paperwork to fire them, get a temporary pharmacist, and initiate a new hiring process to find a permanent replacement.

A consultancy firm offered its services to the VA to help improve the likelihood of hiring a good pharmacist by screening applicants and doing an intensive background check. Suppose the consultants charge a fee for each applicant they screen and are 100% effective in screening out bad applicants (an assumption we will alter in a moment). What is a reasonable fee to pay (let's call it c per applicant screened) for the consultancy firm's work while still saving money for the VA overall?

To solve this problem, we can draw a decision tree for the choice faced by the VA administrator. In this case, we do not have a "finite" decision tree (a tree that ends easily, as in our cancer example in Figure 2.1), but instead we have an "infinite" tree because it is possible that, without a consultant, the administrator would have to fire the first pharmacist, then fire the second one, and so on . . . as shown in Figure 2.3. Each bad pharmacist, as shown in the figure, would prompt a $1,000 firing/rehiring cost, and the whole process would have to start over with another 80% probability of hiring a good pharmacist and a 20% probability of hiring a bad one.

As also shown in Figure 2.3, if the administrator hires a consultant, the VA has to pay a fee ($c/applicant), but bad pharmacists would be identified before hiring, thus

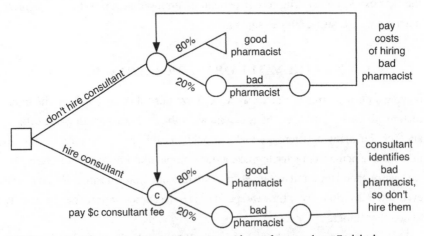

FIGURE 2.3 Decision tree for hiring a pharmacist, with a perfect consultant. Each bad pharmacist would prompt a $1,000 firing/re-hiring cost and the whole process would have to start over with another 80% probability of hiring a good pharmacist and a 20% probability of hiring a bad one. If the administrator hires a consultant, the VA has to pay a fee ($c/applicant), but bad pharmacists would be identified before hiring, preventing the VA from having to pay—when they encounter a bad pharmacist—the extra signing bonus of $50,000 and the extra $1,000 in firing/re-hiring costs.

preventing the VA from having to pay—when they encounter a bad pharmacist—the extra signing bonus of $50,000 and the extra $1,000 in firing/rehiring costs.

We want to know what the value of c would be to make it less costly to hire the consultant than to undergo the hiring process without the consultant. To solve this problem, we can still solve each branch of the decision tree, but our classical approach of "rolling back" from the right side to the root note is made a bit more difficult because we no longer have a classical tree structure. If we wrote out the decision tree as we did for the kidney cancer example, we would have an infinitely long tree because each time we had a bad pharmacist, we would have to draw an extra set of branches. But, for convenience, we have drawn the restarting process as a loop. The loop, however, prevents us from simply solving the tree as we would have in the kidney cancer example.

Suppose we made it easier to solve this problem by defining the expected cost E of hiring a pharmacist as the average cost from many attempts to hire a pharmacist without a consultant (the top main branch of Figure 2.3, labeled "don't hire consultant").

We can see that with probability 0.8, the VA administrator picks a good pharmacist and pays $50,000; with probability 0.2, the administrator picks a bad pharmacist, pays the $50,000, but must also pay $1,000 for a firing/rehiring process. We can write these probabilities and costs as Equation 2.1.

$$E = 0.8 \times \$50,000 + 0.2 \times (\$51,000 + E).$$ [Equation 2.1]

Solving this equation with a little algebra, we find that $E = \$62,750$. In other words, we currently expect that, after the VA administrator tries to hire a bunch of pharmacists, the average cost per pharmacist will be about $62,750 when taking into account the number of pharmacists who are good, the number who are bad, and the cost of firing/rehiring the bad ones.

Next, we can repeat the calculation with the second branch of the decision tree, which is the branch focused on what would happen if the VA administrator hired the consultant. We can define the expected cost F of hiring a pharmacist as the average cost from many attempts to hire a pharmacist after having a consultant on board screening these applicants (the bottom branch of Figure 2.3, labeled "hire consultant").

We can see that the VA administrator has a probability of 0.8 of paying the consultant fee of c and then having a good pharmacist hired with a $50,000 bonus. The administrator also has a probability of 0.2 of paying the consultant fee of c and having a bad pharmacist found by the consultant, who resets the process rather than having the bad pharmacist be hired (saving $51,000 in signing bonus expenses and firing/rehiring fees). If the reset happens, the process of screening starts all over, and the future looks just like it did at the beginning of the problem. We can write these probabilities and costs as Equation 2.2.

$$F = 0.8 \times (c + \$50,000) + 0.2 \times (c + F).$$ [Equation 2.2]

Solving Equation 2.2 for F, we find that the value of F should be $(5/4) \times c + 50000$.

When would the VA want to hire the consultant, if the VA's objective is to save money overall? The consultant would save money overall if F is less than E, meaning that the expected costs with the consultant on board are lower than the expected costs without the consultant on board.

Setting $F < E$ would mean that setting $(5/4) \times c + 50000 < 62,750$. Solving for c, we find that c must be less than $10,200 for the VA to want to hire the consultant.

Here, we've taken information about how often an outcome happens and the costs of that outcome to find the *value of information* or the additional dollars we're willing to spend to avoid a bad outcome. It is possible to apply this type of solution not just to hiring decisions, but to all sorts of public health and healthcare decisions— whether to implement a new test (where the test is the "consultant" helping us to detect a disease), whether to deploy new computer software (which is the "consultant" helping us to improve our workflow), and so on.

In the preceding example, we have solved for the value of *perfect* information because our consultant is perfect at screening out bad apples. But in most cases, we have to solve a value of *imperfect* information problem because the new consultant— or test or computer software that we're considering—is not 100% perfect.

Suppose, for example, that we find that our consultant is not 100% accurate about differentiating good from bad pharmacists. Suppose they have 90% *sensitivity* (see Chapter 1 for definition of this term) for finding bad pharmacists and 80% *specificity* (also see Chapter 1) for finding good pharmacists. In other words, if a pharmacist is bad, then 90% of the time the consultant will say "this one is bad" and the VA administrator starts over and pays for a new applicant's screening process; but 10% of the time, the consultant tells the VA a bad pharmacist is good, and the VA wrongly hires a bad pharmacist. Similarly, if a pharmacist is good, then 80% of the time the consultant will say "this one is good" and hire a good pharmacist; but 20% of the time, the consultant will wrongly say "this one is bad" and the VA starts over and pays for a new applicant's screening process.

We can diagram this new situation by extending our previous decision tree, as shown in Figure 2.4.

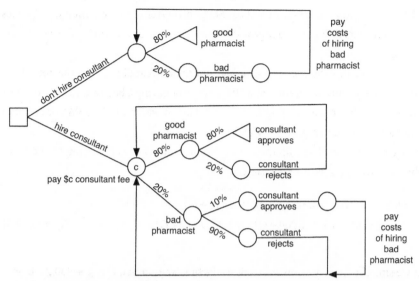

FIGURE 2.4 Decision tree for hiring a pharmacist, with an imperfect consultant. The consultant
has 90% sensitivity for finding bad pharmacists, and 80% specificity for finding good pharmacists.
In other words, if a pharmacist is bad, then 90% of the time the consultant will say "this one is bad"
and the VA administrator starts over and pays for a new applicant's screening process; but 10%
of the time the consultant tells the VA a bad pharmacist is good, and the VA wrongly hires a bad
pharmacist. Similarly, if a pharmacist is good, then 80% of the time the consultant will say "this
one is good' and hire a good pharmacist, but 20% of the time the consultant will wrongly say "this
one is bad" and the VA starts over and pays for a new applicant's screening process.

The top part of our decision tree, the scenario if we don't use the consultant, is the
same as in Figure 2.3. So we only need to solve the bottom part of the tree, which is
the scenario in which the consultant is on board. Here, we can make the problem
simpler to solve by individually solving each of the four possible outcomes (good/
bad pharmacist combined with good/bad consultant decision).

In the first case, the VA has a good pharmacist candidate that the consultant
approves. The VA administrator has an 80% chance of having a good candidate and
an 80% chance that the consultant approves of the candidate, in which case the VA
pays $50,000 and is done with the problem because it had a good outcome.

In the second case, the VA has a good pharmacist candidate that the consultant
rejects. The VA administrator has an 80% chance of having a good candidate and
a 20% chance that the consultant rejects that candidate, in which case the VA goes
back to the starting point to repeat the whole process.

In the third case, the VA has a bad pharmacist candidate that the consultant
approves. The VA administrator has a 20% chance of having a bad candidate and
an 10% chance that the consultant approves of the candidate, in which case the
VA pays $50,000 for the signing bonus and then finds out later that they're a bad

pharmacist and pays an additional $1,000 in firing/rehiring fees. Then the VA goes back to the starting point to repeat the whole process again. This is the worst-case scenario.

In the fourth case, the VA has a bad pharmacist candidate that the consultant rejects. The VA administrator has a 20% chance of having a bad candidate and a 90% chance that the consultant rejects the candidate, in which case the VA goes back to the starting point to repeat the whole process.

We can write and add up these probabilities and costs as Equation 2.3. Let's call the expected costs in this scenario G.

$$G = 0.8 \times 0.8 \times (c + \$50,000) + 0.8 \times 0.2 \times (c + G)$$
$$+ 0.2 \times 0.1 \times (c + \$51,000 + G) + 0.2 \times 0.9 \times (c + G). \qquad \text{[Equation 2.3]}$$

If we simplify this equation with a little algebra, we find that $G = (c + 33020)/0.64$.

Again, we want to find the value of c such that hiring our consultant would be cheaper over all than moving forward without the consultant. So, we solve for the case where $G < E$, or when $(c + 33020)/0.64 < 62{,}750$. Solving for c, we find that our consultant must cost less than $7,140 for us to be willing to pay for their imperfect information.

As we would expect, the value of perfect information ($10,200) is higher than the value of imperfect information ($7,140).

By creating and solving decision trees, we can extend these examples to a variety of situations in which we have new options for preventing disease, screening for disease, or treating disease and need to make wise decisions about whether to pay for the new services, tests, or treatments.

COST-EFFECTIVENESS ANALYSIS

In the previous section, we performed *cost-benefit analysis*, which is the process of synthesizing available information to determine which decision we should make to minimize our overall costs.

In many public health and healthcare decisions, however, our goal is not to minimize overall costs but to spend funds wisely. Even if we spend more money, the benefits in terms of reducing morbidity (cases of disease) and mortality (deaths from disease) may be justified. Typically, we use *cost-effectiveness analysis* to identify how much we reduce disease morbidity or mortality per dollar spent; in contrast to cost-benefit analysis, cost-effectiveness analysis is not just trying to find the strategy with the lowest overall spending, but rather trying to find the strategy that maximizes how much we improve health per each dollar spent.

To illustrate the distinction between these two forms of analysis, suppose we take the example of studying a new therapy for tuberculosis. The standard treatment for tuberculosis in most of the world is prolonged, lasting at least 6 months, and often carries significant side effects for patients. Suppose it costs about $10,000 total. Also suppose a new drug is available that we can add to the standard treatment for tuberculosis. The new drug makes the overall treatment regimen just as effective, but slightly more costly (about $2,000 more for the overall treatment, or $12,000 total). The combined treatment regimen will have more side effects because of the additional drug but will also be shorter, just 4 months. How do we make a fair comparison and evaluate whether this new treatment is "worth" the cost? To put it bluntly: is paying $2,000 more for the treatment "worth" having two months shorter duration of treatment?

The first challenge we face is that the question is no longer purely in terms of dollar amounts: we now have to quantify human suffering, which is an entirely different, and more challenging, enterprise. How do we measure how much less suffering our patients will endure if they have to face side effects for only 4 months instead of 6 months?

One long-standing measure for human suffering is the *quality-adjusted life-year* (QALY; pronounced "qual-ee," as in "quality"), which was devised in the 1960s to create a fair measure of how much suffering people endured from different diseases or treatments.[1] The concept of a QALY is illustrated in Figure 2.5. Suppose that we have a perfectly healthy person and that person lives for 1 year in a state of perfect health: we say that person has gained 1 QALY. Suppose a person is dead in a given

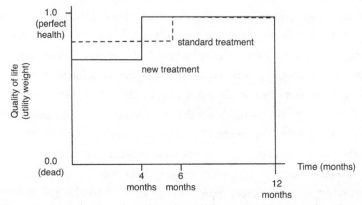

FIGURE 2.5 Conceptualization of a quality-adjusted life-year (QALY), using tuberculosis treatment as an example. The standard treatment is six months and puts people into a moderate state of quality of life (0.8) because of its side-effects. The newer drug that modifies the treatment regimen makes the overall treatment course shorter (four months) but puts people into a lower state of quality of life (0.75) during that period, because of more severe side-effects.

calendar year; that person has gained 0 QALYs. In between the two are most peo-ple with disease, who either are not perfectly healthy (their quality of life, known as their *utility* or *utility weight*, is not a perfect score of 1), or they don't survive for the entire year (the duration of time that they are alive and able to accumulate utility is less than 1 year).

A QALY is therefore a product of two entities: the utility or quality of a person's life in a year and how many years they are in that utility state/at that quality level. Suppose a person is suffering badly from a disease or from side effects of a treat-ment for a short period of time. They may have a low utility (like 0.2 rather than the perfectly healthy utility value of 1) and have that disease for a short period such as 6 months (0.5 of a year), then go back to being perfectly healthy for the rest of the year. Their overall QALYs gained over the year might therefore be 0.2 utility × 0.5 years + 1.0 utility × 0.5 years = 0.6 QALYs gained over the course of the entire year. Suppose, however, that another person has a less-severe disease but that it lasts longer; for example, they may have a moderate utility (like 0.6) but have the disease for the entire year. Their overall QALYs gained over the year would therefore be 0.6 utility × 1 year = 0.6 QALYs. As shown in this example, there is an important caveat to know about QALYs: the overall QALYs accumulated don't provide us with clear information about the disease or treatment. Rather, someone with a brief but severe disease is counted the same way as someone with a less severe but prolonged disease (note that we talk about "discounting" as a strategy to partly address this issue later in the chapter).

Where do utility weight values come from? There are at least four common methods that scientists use to estimate the utility weights for given diseases or treatments.[2] All of these methods utilize surveys of patients with the disease or surveys among people who are healthy but presented with a situation in which they have to make choices about how they would handle a future disease. One type of experiment is known as the "standard gamble" and presents survey respondents with the task of choosing between having a disease for a longer period of time or having a treatment that would either provide them with perfect health or kill them. The worse the disease (the lower the utility weight), the more people are will-ing to risk undergoing the potentially deadly treatment for it rather than staying unhealthy. The standard gamble thus allows scientists to estimate how bad differ-ent diseases are, relative to each other, ranking them from 0 to 1 in terms of utility weights. Another measurement approach is called the "visual analogue scale" and involves asking people with the disease or undergoing a particular treatment with side effects to rate their health from 0 to 100; the score is then divided by 100 to get a utility weight between 0 and 1. The third measurement approach is called a "time tradeoff" study, in which people are asked to theoretically choose between being ill with a given disease (or being on a given treatment for a period of time) or having perfect health for a shorter period but having shorter life-expectancy. As you can imagine, such theoretical experiments are often difficult to believe because people actually experiencing a disease would not be expected to react in the same way as someone imagining a theoretical illness. Furthermore, a person's willingness to undergo various treatments may change over time and with age, as well as from day to day or month to month. Hence, estimating utility values is fundamentally difficult and controversial; important debates have taken place about how to better quantify people's state of health. The fourth and increasingly most common strategy to measure utility is to administer a questionnaire that asks, in a standardized way, about many different domains of life: the ability to participate in daily life activities (such as work and leisure activities), care for oneself (e.g., go to the bathroom or dress oneself without assistance), and be mobile (e.g., walk without pain or shortness of breath). The questionnaire also assesses a person's degree of discomfort or pain, as well as their degree of anxiety or depression. By standardizing such measures, utility values can be calculated similarly across many different diseases or conditions without resorting to theoretical tradeoffs.

Getting back to our tuberculosis example, we can imagine that we can plot out the utility of a person's life while undergoing tuberculosis treatment versus how long they have to undergo treatment, as shown in Figure 2.5.

As shown in Figure 2.5, the utility measure can help us quantify the two key differences between our standard tuberculosis treatment and the new treatment. The standard treatment is 6 months and puts people into a moderate state of quality of life (0.8) because of its side effects. The newer drug that modifies the treatment regimen makes the overall treatment course shorter (4 months) but puts people into a lower state of quality of life (0.75) during that period because of more severe side effects.

From Figure 2.5, we can calculate the expected total number of QALYs under the standard treatment, then under the new treatment.

Under the standard treatment, over the course of 1 year, a patient would gain 0.8 utility × 0.5 year + 1.0 utility × 0.5 year = 0.90 QALYs. Under the new treatment, over the course of 1 year, a patient would gain 0.75 utility × 0.333 year + 1.0 utility × 0.666 year = 0.92 QALYs.

Is this gain in QALYs with the new treatment "worth it"? A typical way of quantifying the value of QALYs gained is to specify the *incremental cost-effectiveness ratio (ICER)*, which is defined in Equation 2.4.

$$ICER = \frac{\left(New\ Cost - Old\ Cost\right)}{\left(New\ QALYs - Old\ QALYs\right)}.$$ [Equation 2.4]

In this case, the ICER is ($12,000 − $10,000)/(0.92 − 0.90) = $100,000 per QALY gained. Is this a good value for money? In prior years, it was common to define that an intervention would be considered "cost-effective" if it cost less than $50,000 per QALY gained.[3] But this threshold has been recognized as inherently arbitrary, particularly because QALYs themselves are so difficult to measure. In more recent years, scientists have tried to identify what different governments or communities are "willing to pay" based on what is actually paid for. Others have argued that a willingness-to-pay threshold should be based on the typical gross domestic product (GDP) of a country, which would potentially discriminate against people in poverty.

Rather than setting an absolute threshold to declare an intervention "cost effective" or "not cost effective," to better inform policy-makers many scientists will now use ICERs to simply compare different interventions and clearly specify whether a treatment is more or less effective, and more or less costly, than an alternative. A common way to differentiate alternative treatments is to plot results on a cost-effectiveness plane, shown in Figure 2.6.

The plane illustrates key terms that we commonly use to define how we interpret the cost-effectiveness of a new treatment compared to an existing one. The x-axis

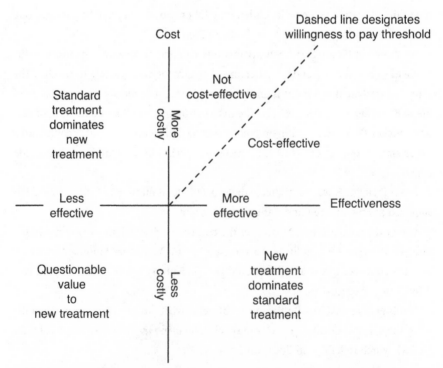

FIGURE 2.6 A cost-effectiveness plane. The x-axis quantifies how effective a treatment is, in quality-adjusted life years (QALYs) or an equivalent metric. The y-axis quantifies how costly the treatment is, in dollars.

quantifies how effective a treatment is in QALYs. The y-axis quantifies how costly the treatment is in dollars. The upper right quadrant is the most common quadrant where we find new treatments: it identifies treatments that are more effective but also more costly. The diagonal line cutting through this quadrant identifies the willingness-to-pay threshold—or how much people are willing to pay for each additional QALY (e.g., $50,000 per QALY, classically). The upper left quadrant is less effective but more costly—a situation in which we say that the standard treatment *dominates* the new treatment; hence, the new treatment is *rejected* or *excluded* (not desirable). The bottom right quadrant is more effective and less costly—a fantastic but rare circumstances in which we say that the new treatment *dominates* the standard treatment; hence, the new treatment should be widely accepted. Finally, the bottom left quadrant indicates when a treatment is less effective but also less costly. Most of the time such a treatment would be questionable at best because we wouldn't want to save money at the expense of causing more morbidity or mortality.

COMMON TERMS AND METRICS

Sometimes scientists will use the term *cost-utility analysis* to refer to the type of analysis we just performed, in which we calculated an ICER in terms of dollars spent per QALY gained. The concept is meant to highlight that we have incorporated utility values into our analysis. These scientists might strictly refer to cost-effectiveness analysis as a situation in which we do not adjust the life-years gained with utility values, but simply analyze total life-years gained from one treatment versus another. The problem with such a cost-effectiveness analysis is that it only looks at gains in life expectancy, not in whether that life expectancy gain is painful and full of suffering or healthy and happy. Often the term "cost-effectiveness analysis" is applied widely without clarifying that most cost-effectiveness analyses in the literature are actually cost-utility analyses because they take into account QALYs rather than absolute numbers of years of life gained.

Similarly, other critics will choose to tabulate the utility value of a treatment in terms of *disability-adjusted life-years* (DALYs; pronounced "dah-lees") rather than QALYs. DALYs are conceptually different from QALYs because they focus on a loss rather than a gain: DALYs focus on how much life is lost due to disability and early death from a disease. Therefore, a good intervention will reduce the number of DALYs lost to a disease. While QALYs are calculated as a utility value times the number of years lived at that utility value, DALYs are calculated as the sum of two components, as shown in Equation 2.5.

DALYs = Years of Life Lost + Years of Life Lived with Disability.   [Equation 2.5]

Years of life lost is calculated per Equation 2.6.

Years of Life Lost = Number of deaths due to condition
$$\times \text{ (Life expectancy} - \text{Age of death from condition).}$$

[Equation 2.6]

Years of life lived with disability is calculated per Equation 2.7.

Years of life lived with disability = Incidence of disease in population
$$\times \text{ Disability weight for the disease}$$
$$\times \text{ Duration of the disease until remission or death.}$$

[Equation 2.7]

In older tabulations, DALYs were often calculated by including different disability (disutility) weights for different age groups, such that losses of life from older adults were not counted as heavily as those among younger adults.[4] This practice became controversial and is no longer commonly done.[5]

DALYs are currently used by the World Health Organization to help tally the burden of disease in an overall population and therefore how much an intervention reduces the burden of disease in an overall population, rather than just for a single individual. The practice brings up the issue of *perspective* in cost-effectiveness analyses, which refers to the idea that, for any given analysis in which we are tabulating costs and/or effectiveness (using any measure such as QALYs or DALYs), we have to define who we are doing the analysis *for*. For example, an individual person in the United Kingdom may not pay many of the costs of their medical treatment because those costs typically are covered by the UK National Health Service (with the caveat that the person indirectly pays through taxes to the government, which then pools the funds). But most cost-effectiveness analyses are performed from the "societal" perspective, which means that—regardless of who pays—we wish to know as a society how much is being gained in paying for a new test, intervention, or treatment and how much is being gained. Some analyses may nevertheless be made from other perspectives, such as the perspective of an individual government agency or an insurance company.

Finally, a common practice in cost-effectiveness analysis is to "discount" both the costs and QALY/DALY estimates tabulated in a cost-effectiveness analysis. *Discounting* or *temporal discounting* refers to the finding in behavioral economics in which people tend to value money and health in the short-term more than they value money and health in the long-term. For example, most people choose to receive $100 immediately rather than receiving $100 1 month from now, even though both choices are worth the same amount of money. To take into account the fact that people tend to favor immediate money savings or immediate health gains more than distant ones, cost-effectiveness analyses typically tend to discount each year of costs or QALYs taken into account in an analysis by a small factor (usually around 3% by convention), per Equation 2.8.

Current value = Future value / [(1 + discount rate) ∧ (years in the future)].

[Equation 2.8]

For example, if applying a 3% annual discount rate to a calculation of costs, a therapy that costs \$100 next year will be calculated as costing \$100/(1.03^1) = \$97, as compared to a therapy that costs \$100 this year, which will remain valued at \$100 in present-day dollars. Similarly, a therapy that prevents disease 5 years in the future and gains 0.1 QALYs in 5 years would be worth 0.1/(1.03^5) = 0.09 QALYs in present-day terms as compared to a therapy that saves 0.1 QALYs this year and remains valued at 0.1 QALYs. Typically, cost-effectiveness studies tend to calculate and sum all costs and QALYs over a long-term "time horizon," usually the overall life expectancy of a person, to compare all costs and health states in the future. But discounting has been controversial because it may undervalue the benefits of preventative interventions and favor short-term therapies instead.[6]

3

OPTIMIZATION

In this chapter, we seek to answer the question: how can we best allocate limited resources among many different programs? Suppose we are given a budget to run a program, but we need to distribute that budget among many different alternative projects; for example, within a public health department, we might allocate some resources (personnel, money, equipment) to a vaccination program, another set of resources to a diabetes prevention program, and yet another set of resources to an air pollution reduction program. How can we try to maximize the chances that we allocate limited resources fairly, ensuring that each program has at least the minimal resources that it needs while also ensuring that the distribution of resources maximizes overall public health? In Chapter 1, we derived a simple model of resource allocation in which we allocated inspectors to different food processing factories; yet, in most circumstances, we have more than one resource (not just personnel) to distribute among more than one or two types of sites or programs (not just high- vs. low-risk factories). Very quickly, solving such a problem becomes unwieldy if we attempt to solve it as a simple linear expression, as we did in Chapter 1. In this chapter, we will use computational tools to solve such problems for us. The problems we will address are fundamentally different from the cost-benefit or cost-effectiveness analyses we solved in Chapter 2. Rather than evaluating how much we should pay for a resource (a test, treatment, or intervention) or whether a particular resource is cost-effective, this chapter focuses on how we can make smart decisions to maximize the potential effectiveness or cost-effectiveness of any particular program we're interested in supporting—a goal known as *optimization*.

THE MECHANICS OF BUDGET OPTIMIZATION

Suppose that we live in a city that has two beaches, beach A and beach B. Also suppose that we have been put in charge of allocating lifeguards between these two beaches. The lifeguards have all received their training and certification, and each lifeguard costs only $100 per summer in salary and equipment costs (what a good deal!).

Our goal is to save as many lives as possible this summer by allocating the life-guards between the two beaches in a distribution that maximizes the total number of people who would be prevented from drowning. The total number of people who would be prevented from drowning cannot be known in advance, of course; hence, the best we can do is use historical data to inform our understanding of which beach might be more dangerous and how many people, typically, were saved from near-drowning episodes on each beach, based on how many lifeguards were placed on that beach in previous years.

By searching in the historical town archives, we were able to calculate the expected (average) number of near-drowning episodes averted each summer based on data from the past decade. These data are summarized in Table 3.1.

To clarify Table 3.1, the first row specifies that if no lifeguards were on either beach, then—unsurprisingly—no near-drowning episodes were averted. The second row specifies that if 1 lifeguard was on beach A, then, on average, 2 near-drowning episodes were averted on beach A (2 lives saved). If 1 lifeguard was on beach B, then, on average, 1 near-drowning episode was averted on beach B (1 life saved). Similarly, per the last row, if 3 lifeguards were on beach A, then 4 lives were saved, on average, on beach A. If 3 lifeguards were on beach B, then 5 lives were saved, on average, on beach B.

The concept of *diminishing returns* is evident from Table 3.1. With an increasing number of lifeguards on each beach, there often is a decreasing benefit (thinking mathematically, the slope of the line between number of lifeguards and number of lives saved has a lower slope with each additional lifeguard). This is often the case for resource allocation because the first or second lifeguard on a beach may be very helpful, but adding a third lifeguard when there are already two lifeguards may not make as much difference.

Here is our challenge: our city has not decided how much money it wants to invest in lifeguards for this summer. The city council could conceivably spend up to $300 this summer, which would be enough to hire three lifeguards overall to spread between the two beaches.

Table 3.1 The expected (average) number of near-drowning episodes averted each summer based on data from the past decade

Number of lifeguards put on beach	Expected (average number of) lives saved given number of lifeguards put on beach A	Expected (average number of) lives saved given number of lifeguards put on beach B
0	0	0
1	2	1
2	3	4
3	4	5

Suppose we wanted to find out how to maximize the number of lives we would save this summer depending on what budget we were given—from $100 to $200 to $300 total for the summer.

How would we go about distributing the lifeguards we could hire at each level of budget?

One strategy for solving this problem is to draw out each possible choice as a node in a decision tree. In other words, if we are given $100, what's the best place to put one life guard? If we are given $200, what's the best place to put a second lifeguard? And, finally, if we are given $300, what's the best place to put our third lifeguard? In each stage of the decision tree, we are effectively calculating the *marginal returns* from each additional lifeguard, meaning the incremental benefit we get from an incremental increase in resources.

Let's start in Figure 3.1 with a decision tree showing the marginal returns of increasing from zero lifeguards to one lifeguard (a total budget of $100) for either beach.

To prevent confusion in our accounting, we will keep track of the lives saved in our decision tree by labeling each node with the number saved on beach A plus the number saved on beach B. For example, if we write "save 2 + 1 lives" above a node, it means we expect to save 2 lives on beach A and 1 life on beach B for a total of 3 lives saved over the summer.

As shown in Figure 3.1, we'd expect to save 2 lives if our first guard was placed on beach A and only 1 life if our first guard was placed on beach B (reading row 3 of Table 3.1). But we shouldn't jump to the conclusion that it means all further guards should be on beach A or that only the first branch of the decision tree should be pursued. It's worthwhile to flesh out the full decision tree to see what possible outcomes could result with the next guard and the third guard. Figure 3.2 illustrates our

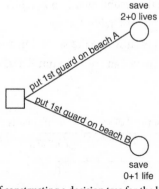

FIGURE 3.1 The first stage of constructing a decision tree for the lifeguard distribution problem, showing the marginal returns of increasing from zero lifeguards to one lifeguard (a total budget of $100) for either beach.

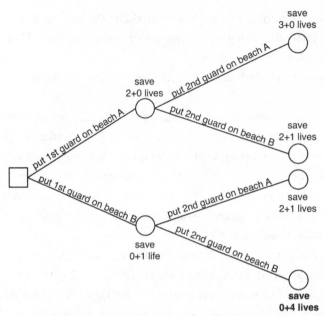

FIGURE 3.2 The second stage of constructing a decision tree for the lifeguard distribution problem, showing our options for where to place a second guard, if our total budget increased from $100 to $200.

options for where to place a second guard if our total budget increased from $100 to $200.

We can read Figure 3.2 from the top to bottom branch. As shown in Figure 3.2, we'd expect that if we put the first guard on beach A and the second guard on beach A, we'd save 3 lives at beach A (row 4 of Table 3.1). If we put the first guard on beach A and the second guard on beach B, we'd save 2 lives from the first guard on beach A (row 3 of Table 3.1) and an additional 1 life from the one guard we've now put on beach B (row 3 of Table 3.1), for a total of 3 lives saved. If we put the first guard on beach B and the second guard on beach A, we'd save 2 lives on beach A and 1 life on beach B (row 3 of Table 3.2), for a total of 3 lives saved. Finally, if we put the first guard on beach B and the second guard on beach B, we'd save 4 lives (row 4 of Table 3.2). So we can see from our decision tree that there are four

Table 3.2 Final tally of optimal distribution of lifeguards among beaches

Budget	Lifeguards at A	Lifeguards at B	Total lives saved
$100	1	0	2
$200	0	2	4
$300	1	2	6

equivalent options for what to do with $200; no matter what path we take, we'd expect to save 4 lives over the summer.

Hence, if we only have $200 for the summer, we should place both guards on beach B. As shown in this illustration, we should have pursued the top left branch of the tree if we only had $100, but it was important to keep open the bottom left branch of the tree to get the best solution once the budget was increased.

Naturally, the next step for determining how to allocate the last $100, for a total budget of $300 over the summer, is illustrated by extending our decision tree one step further, as drawn in Figure 3.3.

Reading from the top to the bottom branch of Figure 3.3, we can conduct a final tally of all possible outcomes. The topmost branch involves putting the first guard on beach A and the second guard on beach A; adding the third guard to beach A would lead to four lives saved (row 5 of Table 3.1), while adding the third guard to beach B would lead to 3 lives saved on beach A and 1 life saved on beach B (by virtue of having 2 guards on beach A and 1 guard on beach B).

The next cluster of two branches starts from the trunk of putting the first guard on beach A followed by the branch of putting the second guard on beach B; adding

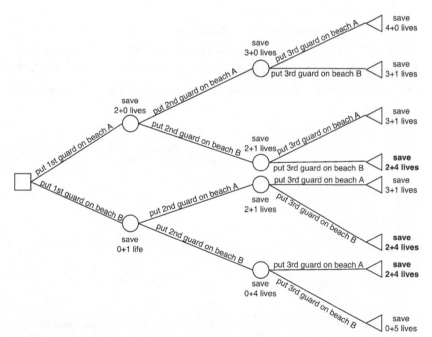

FIGURE 3.3 The third and final stage of constructing a decision tree for the lifeguard distribution problem, showing our options for where to place a third guard, if our total budget increased from $200 to $300. We have mapped out all possibilities, and we see that there are three optimal ways to spend $300, put in bold in the Figure. In all cases, the best way to spend $300 is to put 1 guard on beach A and 2 guards on beach B.

the third guard to beach A would save 3 lives on beach A and 1 on beach B (because a total of 2 guards would be on beach A [row 4 of Table 3.2] and 1 guard on beach B [row 3 of Table 3.2]). Alternatively adding a third guard to beach B would result in 1 guard on A and 2 guards on B, for a total of 6 lives saved (2 from beach A and 4 from beach B). So far, this is our best possible outcome.

The third cluster of two branches starts from the trunk of putting the first guard on beach B followed by the branch of putting the second guard on beach A. Adding a third guard on beach A would result in 3 lives saved on beach A and 1 on beach B (due to 2 guard on A and 1 guard on B). Alternatively putting the third guard on B would result in 1 guard on A and 2 guards on B for a total of 2 lives saved from beach A and 4 from beach B.

Finally, the bottom cluster of branches starts from the trunk of putting the first guard on beach B followed by the branch of putting the second guard on beach B. If we put the third guard on beach A, we would save 6 lives (2 from A and 4 from B). If we put the third guard on B, we would save 5 lives (all on beach B).

Hence, we have mapped out all possibilities in Figure 3.3, and we see that there are three optimal ways to spend $300, shown in bold in the figure. In all cases, the best way to spend $300 is to put 1 guard on beach A and 2 guards on beach B.

We summarize our results in Table 3.2.

A graph of this solution is shown in Figure 3.4.

In more formal terms, we have solved a problem in which we have an *objective function*, which is defined as a function of our choices that we seek to maximize, minimize, or set to a particular value. In our case, the objective function is the

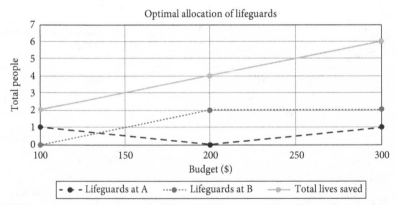

FIGURE 3.4 Optimal allocation in the lifeguard distribution problem. The x-axis shows the total budget available, in increasing increments of $100. The y-axis shows the total number of people: optimal number of guards on beach A, optimal number of guards on beach B, and people whose lives are saved with the optimal budget allocation, at each incremental increase in the total budget from $100 to $300.

number of lives saved across both beaches. If $b_i(x_i)$ represents the total benefits in terms of lives saved that we achieve from putting x_i lifeguards at the ith beach (here, i equals A or B), where x_i must be integers greater than or equal to zero, then we have sought to maximize the objective function $b_A(x_A) + b_B(x_B)$.

Solving an objective function is generally subject to a *budgetary constraint*, which we can call **B**. In our case, the budgetary constraint totaled either $100, $200, or $300, and we can write that the budgetary constraint equation was $100x_A + 100x_B \leq$ **B**.

SPREADSHEET-BASED OPTIMIZATION

Our lifeguard problem provided us with a general template for solving optimization problems. Given information about how effective a resource is when allocated in one way or another, we can create a decision tree to maximize the expected benefits from allocating the resources within a given budget.

Yet our simple lifeguard problem produced a relatively large decision tree despite calling for the allocation of just one resource (lifeguards) among just two entities (two beaches) with just one constraint (the budget). For many problems of resource allocation, we have many resources we could distribute, with many entities to distribute among, and many constraints (not just budgetary, but also regulatory requirements, internal company requirements, community desires, and so on). Drawing all of these possibilities as a decision tree would be arduous and inefficient.

Hence, for problems that involve potentially complex decision trees, we can resort to using our computational resources instead of solving the problems by hand.

Suppose we encounter the following problem: we are running a charity-based primary care clinic for a low-income community, and we need to decide our schedule for offering clinical services. Suppose we have 10 sessions of clinical services to schedule per week because our clinic is open 5 days a week and is organized into half-day sessions. There are three types of activities we need to offer at our clinic: primary care services (i.e., routine patient visits), vaccination services, and cancer screening services (Pap screens for cervical cancer). Our challenge is to decide how many half-day sessions to offer for each of these activities.

Suppose that our objective is to maximize the number of quality-adjusted life-years (QALYs) that we save among our patient population, subject to a number of constraints. Table 3.3 reveals the number of QALYs that each activity saves per week among our patient population. The table also provides information on the equipment costs for each half-day session (with Pap screens costing the most because of their material costs) and on the labor costs per session in terms of how much you have to pay the staff given the different staff needed for each type of session.

Table 3.3 The number of QALYs that each activity saves per week among our patient population

	Type of session		
	Primary care	Vaccination	Pap screening
QALYs gained per session	0.08	0.02	0.04
Equipment cost per session	$100	$30	$200
Personnel cost per session	$75	$25	$300

QALY, quality-adjusted life-years.

As shown in Table 3.3, primary care is most helpful for our patient population in this example in terms of the number of QALYs saved per session offered. But we cannot just offer primary care services because there are several other constraints that we need to fulfill. As a charity clinic, we have a limited budget for equipment and a second budget limit for personnel. Furthermore, we need to offer at least one session per week of each of the three types of services and fill the full 5-day week with a total of 10 half-day sessions. These constraints and requirements are summarized in Table 3.4.

If we created a decision tree to solve this problem, we would quickly be overwhelmed because there would be three branches for the first half-day session of the week (one branch if we allocated the session to primary care, a second branch for vaccination, and a third for Pap screening) and another set of three branches for the second half-day session ... continuing onward to the tenth branch for the tenth half-day session of the week, producing 3^{10} or 59,049 branches. At each branch, we would need to calculate how much we spent so far on equipment, on personnel, and what the total number of QALYs saved was at that point. We would then need

Table 3.4 Service constraints and requirements for a charity clinic

Description	Constraint
Equipment budget	$1,030
Personnel budget	$925
Minimum number of primary care half-day sessions/week	1
Minimum number of vaccination half-day sessions/week	1
Minimum number of Pap screen half-day sessions/week	1
Number of half-day sessions that must be offered per week	10

to search for the branches that gave us the most QALYs while fulfilling all of the requirements.

A simpler approach is to put all of our information into a spreadsheet and allow a spreadsheet program such as Microsoft Excel to find the optimal decision tree pathway for us. The spreadsheet corresponding to this problem can be downloaded from this book's website (https://github.com/sanjaybasu/modelinghealthsystems/). On the spreadsheet, we can see that several tables have been created based on Tables 3.3 and 3.4. Figure 3.5 also illustrates the spreadsheet.

In our spreadsheet, we have laid out the optimization problem by having the key decision at the top: in this case, the number of clinic sessions we hope to devote to primary care, vaccination, or Pap screening services are in the first row of the table

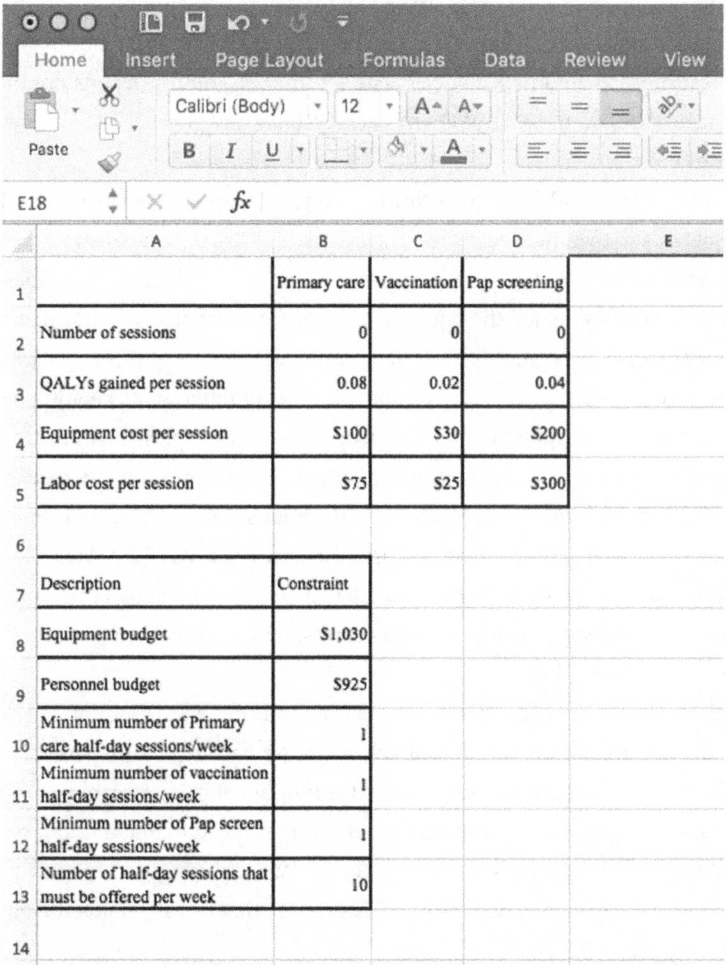

	A	B	C	D	E
1		Primary care	Vaccination	Pap screening	
2	Number of sessions	0	0	0	
3	QALYs gained per session	0.08	0.02	0.04	
4	Equipment cost per session	$100	$30	$200	
5	Labor cost per session	$75	$25	$300	
6					
7	Description	Constraint			
8	Equipment budget	$1,030			
9	Personnel budget	$925			
10	Minimum number of Primary care half-day sessions/week	1			
11	Minimum number of vaccination half-day sessions/week	1			
12	Minimum number of Pap screen half-day sessions/week	1			
13	Number of half-day sessions that must be offered per week	10			
14					

FIGURE 3.5 Illustration of the clinic scheduling optimization problem, solved in Microsoft Excel. The spreadsheet corresponding to this problem can be downloaded from this book's website.

in the spreadsheet. The values in the first row of data are set to 0 for starters—or, alternatively, to any guess we might have for the optimal number of clinic sessions for each of the three activities. Later, we will have Excel find the right combination of sessions for us; hence, the current values are just placeholders.

The next few rows in the spreadsheet provide the input data from Table 3.3, providing Excel with the key data our computer needs to identify the QALY benefits and costs associated with each clinic session.

The final few rows consist of our constraints, listed in Table 3.4.

The critical task ahead of us is to calculate how we will fulfill all of our constraints while maximizing the number of QALYS saved by our clinic. To achieve this task, we have to input equations into our spreadsheet that allow us to relate the number of half-day clinical sessions we are allocating among each of the three activities to the numbers of QALYs and costs created by these sessions. In other words, we need to set up the spreadsheet to make use of the information we have put in. We want the spreadsheet to automatically calculate whether all the constraints are met and to calculate the total number of QALYs achieved for any given choice of how many sessions to offer.

To set up the spreadsheet to perform the key calculations, we have to insert several equations so that the spreadsheet can calculate whether each constraint has been met given the number of sessions being chosen for each of the three activities.

The first equation is for the equipment budget constraint. We can calculate the equipment spending by multiplying the number of sessions of primary care by the equipment cost per primary care session, plus the number of vaccination sessions multiplied by the equipment cost per vaccination session, plus the number of Pap screening sessions multiplied by the equipment cost per Pap screening session. In Figure 3.5 and our example spreadsheet on the book's website, the equation is in cell D8, and we have typed into that cell the equation "=B2*B4+C2*C4+D2*D4." The equals sign means that we want Excel to calculate something (in this case, how much we're spending on equipment); the letters correspond to the column and numbers to the row of the spreadsheet.

Similarly, the second equation is for the personnel budget constraint. We can calculate the personnel spending in cell D9, where we have typed the personnel costs of each primary care session multiplied by the number of primary care sessions, plus the personnel costs of each vaccination session multiplied by the number of vaccination sessions, plus the personnel costs of each Pap screening session multiplied by the number of Pap screening sessions. This means that cell D9 holds the equation "=B2*B5+C2*C5+D2*D5."

The next set of constraints are those specifying that we need to provide the minimum number of clinic sessions for each type of clinic. Hence, in cells D10, D11, and

D12, we have entered "=B2," "=C2," and "=D2," respectively; this provides us with the value of the current number of clinic sessions to compare against our required number of sessions.

The last constraint is the number of sessions offered per week, which must be equal to 10 sessions. The current number of sessions is calculated in cell D13, which holds the equation "=B2+C2+D2."

As shown in the spreadsheet and in Figure 3.6, we have inserted symbols in column C, rows 8 through 13, to specify whether our calculated value for budget and session numbers must be greater than or equal to, less than or equal to, or equal to our constraint. For example, the calculated value for the equipment budget must be less than or equal to $1,030, and the calculated value for the total number of sessions per week must be equal to 10. Excel doesn't read this text; it is simply there for us to keep track of our constraints.

Finally, we have to insert our objective function: the number of QALYs per week, which we are trying to maximize. The number of QALYs saved per week is the number of primary care sessions multiplied by the QALYs saved per primary care session, plus the number of vaccination sessions multiplied by the QALYs saved per vaccination session, plus the number of Pap screening sessions multiplied by the QALYs saved per Pap screening session. The number of QALYs per week is inserted into cell D14, where we have typed "=B2*B3+C2*C3+D2*D3."

Now that we have set up our spreadsheet to automatically calculate the budgets, sessions offered, and QALYs from any choice we make for the number of sessions, we can manually look at what combinations of primary care, vaccination, and Pap screening sessions would produce different budgetary and QALY results. For example, if we replaced the first row of data (row 2) with the choice of 1 primary care session per week, 3 vaccination sessions per week, and 5 Pap screening sessions per week, we can see that our spreadsheet instantly calculates the equipment budget as $1,190, the personnel budget as $1,650, and the QALYs saved per week as 0.34. Unfortunately, we see that our budget is already too high for the budget constraints.

Rather than undertaking a repeated trial-and-error process to find the best combination of sessions, we can have Excel find the optimal number of sessions for us. Excel uses the "Solver" algorithm, which effectively draws the complex decision tree for us and finds the optimal branch to follow to ensure that our objective function is maximized within the constraints that we set. To turn on the Solver algorithm, we go to "Tools," select "Add-ins," and ensure the Solver box is checked (those without a Solver option may need to upgrade to a more advanced version of Excel).

Once the algorithm is activated, select "Tools" and "Solver" and a pop-up window will appear that looks similar to Figure 3.7. Although different versions of Excel

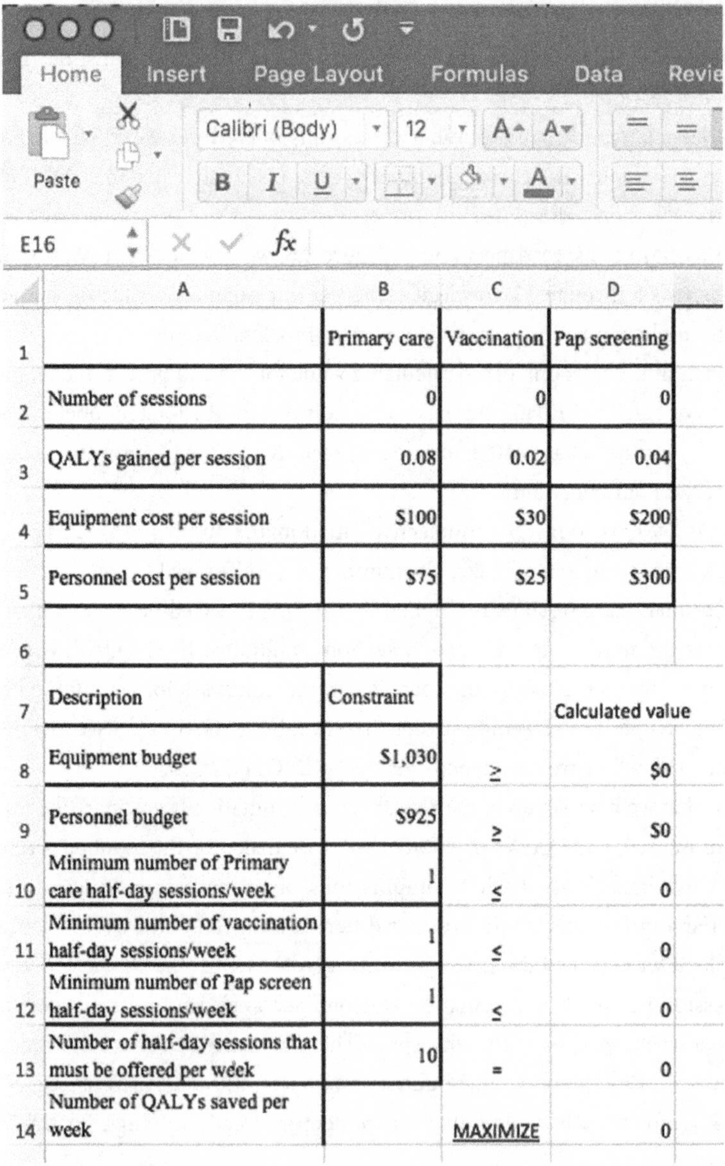

	A	B	C	D
1		Primary care	Vaccination	Pap screening
2	Number of sessions	0	0	0
3	QALYs gained per session	0.08	0.02	0.04
4	Equipment cost per session	$100	$30	$200
5	Personnel cost per session	$75	$25	$300
6				
7	Description	Constraint		Calculated value
8	Equipment budget	$1,030	≥	$0
9	Personnel budget	$925	≥	$0
10	Minimum number of Primary care half-day sessions/week	1	≤	0
11	Minimum number of vaccination half-day sessions/week	1	≤	0
12	Minimum number of Pap screen half-day sessions/week	1	≤	0
13	Number of half-day sessions that must be offered per week	10	=	0
14	Number of QALYs saved per week		MAXIMIZE	0

FIGURE 3.6 Illustration of the clinic scheduling optimization problem, solved in Microsoft Excel. The number of QALYs per week is inserted into cell D14, where we have typed "=B2*B3+C2*C3+D2*D3".

show a different layout or appearance to the Solver algorithm, they all contain the same basic functionality.

The first cell we have to complete is the objective function or "set objective" cell. That is cell D14, the total DALYs we hope to save. We select that we want to "Max," or maximize, the value of this cell.

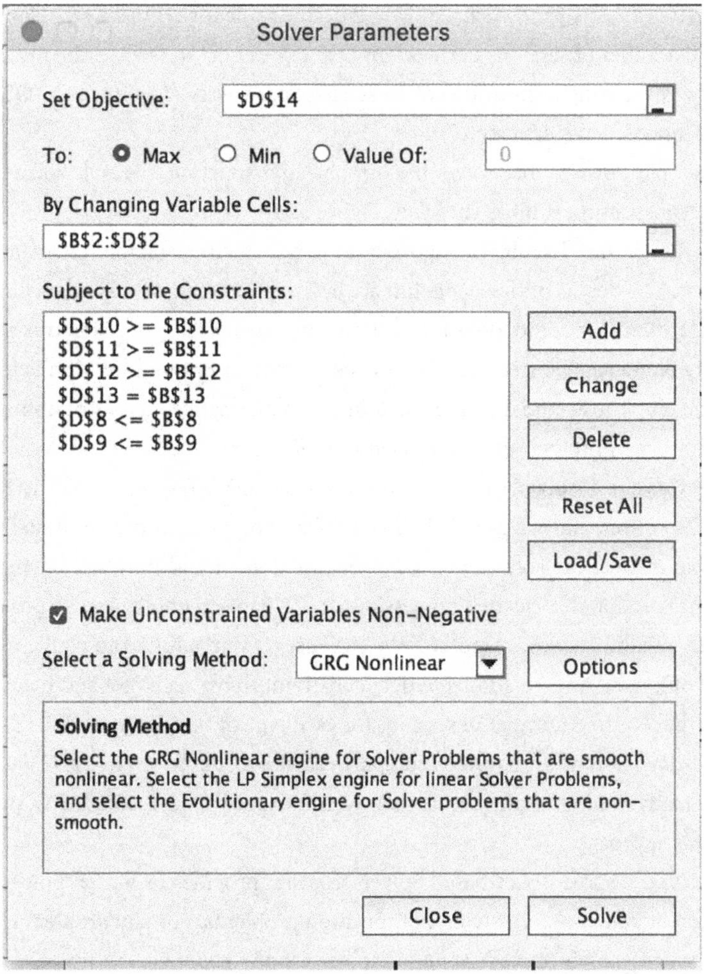

FIGURE 3.7 **Solver window for the clinic scheduling optimization problem, solved in Microsoft Excel.**

We next have to specify which cells we want Excel to change in order to maximize our objective function. In our case, it's the cells that correspond to the number of clinic sessions per week: cells B2, C2, and D2. We can insert this by typing B2:D2 in the "by changing variable cells" box.

Next, we have to add the constraints that we want to fulfill. We click "Add" to add each constraint individually. We first add that we want our calculated budget value in cell D8 to be less than or equal to the constraint of the equipment budget typed into cell B8. We put D8 as the "cell reference" to be "<=" the "constraint" B8, and click "Add." Similarly, we put the calculated personnel budget value in cell D9 to be "<=" the constraint B9, and click add. We then put the days of primary care sessions in D10 to be greater than or equal to (switch the middle button to show a ">=" symbol) the constraint in B10 and click "Add," and do the same for D11 and D12. Finally, we have the number of sessions per week in D13 to be equal to (switch the middle button to "=") the constraint in B13 of 10 sessions per week. We then click "OK" to go back to the main Solver screen.

We should now see that Solver has our objective function, the cells it can change, and the constraints set up as shown in Figure 3.7.

We will use the default solving method here, which is suitable for most of our problems. The details of the algorithm are beyond the scope of this book, but, effectively, the solving method looks for the best path down a large decision tree and tests a variety of alternative tree branches to ensure that an optimal solution is found to our problem. Those students interested in the mathematical details of optimization algorithms can find their details derived in R. K. Arora (2015).[1]

When we click "Solve," the program should take just a few seconds to arrive at an optimal solution, and we can click "Keep Solver Solution" to return to our spreadsheet and inspect the solution. The Solver function should find that having 8 primary care sessions, 1 vaccination session, and 1 Pap screening session per week is the optimal allocation of resources. We can inspect our solution to confirm that all of our equipment and personnel budget constraints have been met and that we have offered the required number of sessions for each type of activity, as well as filled all of our half-day sessions as required (compare cells B8 through B13 to cells D8 through D13). Finally, our solution reveals that we can expect to save 0.7 QALYs per week using this approach.

Overall, the spreadsheet-based Solver program provides us with a powerful and easily extendable tool for solving optimization problems. For any problem in which we can specify an objective function that we wish to maximize, minimize, or set to a particular value, we can specify what factors are in our control and what constraints we have to meet. Under these constraints, Solver should be able to find a solution (if a solution exists) to optimize our decision, fulfill the constraints, and save us the effort of creating a very large decision tree that would often be unwieldy to sort through by hand.

PART TWO

Operations

4

WAITING LINES AND WAITING TIMES

In this chapter, we seek to answer the question: how can we reduce the time it takes to deliver a public health or healthcare service? Suppose we have a program for which the supply of personnel, equipment, or other resources is exceeded by the demand for services. This often occurs in public health and healthcare, which is why we have long waiting times in emergency departments, long waiting lists for under-supported services such as drug rehabilitation, and vast periods of uncertainty for scarce commodities such as organ transplants. How can we minimize the time it takes to provide people with the services they need? Embedded in this question is the problem of how we can make strategic decisions about distributing our resources, such as whether hiring a new nurse or buying a new piece of equipment will decrease the time it takes to deliver a service. Should we invest in that new resource, or is our money better spent on something else? In this chapter, we will solve such problems using a common operations research method known as *queuing systems*, which are systems of equations that enable us to determine what factors influence the time people are in a waiting line (or queue, if you're British). We'll first learn about how to calculate waiting times and interpret rates of service delivery, then develop two common equations that we can use to determine how much that changes to our resource allocation decisions will affect waiting times and the number of people waiting in those lines.

UNDERSTANDING RATES

To understand waiting times, we first need to have a good understanding of epidemiological *rates*. By definition, a rate refers to a description of the number of people or objects per unit time—such as 10 people per hour eating in a café or 20 cars per minute traveling through an intersection.

To really understand how to translate estimates of "rates" into estimates of "waiting times" for public health models, we can start with a silly example. Suppose you are a businessperson who manages a warehouse business. Your warehouse stores and

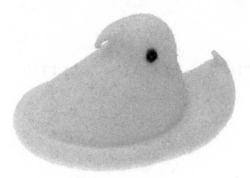

FIGURE 4.1 **Peeps.**

supplies Peeps—those brightly colored marshmallow candies that appear in trick-or-treat containers every Halloween (Figure 4.1).

First of all, shame on you for giving little children excess sugar!

But that problem aside, suppose you want to be a savvy businessperson and optimize your warehouse business. Your business is based on the premise that you need to buy a certain number of Peeps from the manufacturer and sell a certain number of Peeps to grocery stores who buy the products from you, hopefully providing you with a profit.

As a savvy businessperson, you know that you shouldn't order too many Peeps from the manufacturer and have them sitting on the shelf for weeks or months because you'll be wasting your money shelving a product rather than selling it. On the other hand, you also know that you shouldn't order too few Peeps from the manufacturer because the grocery store will want more, and you effectively lose money if you can't meet the high demand. Your business model can be captured in a simple diagram, shown in Figure 4.2.

To determine the optimal number of Peeps to order from the manufacturer to satisfy your marshmallow-craving customer base, you need to figure out the demand that people are placing on your warehouse. Suppose you do a simple survey at your warehouse, in which you ask your manager: "How long does the average Peep stay on the shelf in my warehouse before it gets ordered and shipped off to the grocery store?"

The manufacturer can tag some Peeps with a label as soon as they come from the manufacturer and can keep track of how many days it takes before the labeled Peeps

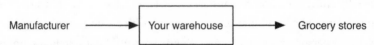

FIGURE 4.2 **Illustration of a business model that involves two rates:** a rate of purchasing product from the manufacturer, and a rate of selling product from your warehouse to the grocery store.

leave your warehouse shelf and get shipped to grocery stores. Suppose the average Peep, according to this experiment, stays on the shelf 3 days. In that case, what is the average *per Peep rate* of leaving the warehouse?

We can say that 1 Peep lasts on average 3 days, hence the average per Peep rate of leaving the warehouse is 1 Peep/3 days = 1/3 of a Peep per day. Here, we can see that, for rates of transfer, we have a value of time that is in the denominator of our equation, which is why epidemiological rates are often confusing—they typically have units such as days⁻¹ or 1/days, which simply means that they are reflecting some change per unit time.

Suppose that, instead of having each Peep last for 3 days, you have a sudden surge in business because it's the week before Halloween. Peeps are flying off of your shelves at a rate of five Peeps per day on average. What's the average *survival time* of one Peep on your warehouse shelf?

We can say that the survival time is 1 day for each set of 5 Peeps, or 1/5 of a day of survival time on the shelf of the warehouse.

To generalize, we see that the duration of time that a Peep survives on the warehouse shelf is the inverse of the duration of time it spent on the shelf. Equation 4.1 provides the general nomenclature for this relationship.

$$E(T) = \frac{1}{\mu}.$$
[Equation 4.1]

In this equation $E(T)$ refers to the expected (or average) duration of the time T that a Peep survives on the shelf in your warehouse, and μ is the average per Peep rate of leaving the warehouse, also known as the *removal rate*. Hence, the duration of time spent in a given state is the inverse of the rate of leaving that state. For example, the duration of life (a.k.a., life expectancy) is the inverse of the rate of death (the mortality rate). As another example, suppose the average time that a Peep stays on your warehouse shelf is 0.2 days. From Equation 4.1, $E(T) = 0.2$ days. How many Peeps should you order from the factory per day to perfectly meet the demand? Using the formula to calculate the rate of Peeps leaving the warehouse, you can estimate that you need to deliver Peeps at a rate of 1/0.2, or 5 Peeps/day. Hence, you should order 5 Peeps per day, on average, to keep up with the demand.

Of course, all of these expressions are just averages. Suppose we want to come up with a way of determining what the probability is that a Peep "survives" on the shelf for 1 day, or 2 days, or 15 days. Then we need to find a function to describe the probability that a Peep stays on your warehouse shelf for at least t units of time. We can write that as $\Pr\{T > t\}$, or the probability that a Peep's survival time T is greater than some value t. This is a type of *survival function*, designated $S(t)$.

How can we derive such a function? We can reason that the average shelf life in the warehouse, $E(T)$, is a sum of 1 day*Pr{Peep on shelf 1st day} + 1day*Pr{Peep still on shelf 2nd day} + 1day*Pr{peep still on shelf 3rd day} + · · · all the way to infinity days (by which time, presumably, the probability of surviving on the shelf has reached 0). In other words, our average shelf life $E(T)$ is the sum of Pr{$T > t$} across all possible values of t. We want to find some survival function $S(t)$ for which this is true. Writing down this expression, we have Equation 4.2:

$$E(T) = \int_0^\infty \Pr\{T > t\}dt \ = \ \int_0^\infty S(t)dt \ = \frac{1}{\mu}. \qquad \text{[Equation 4.2]}$$

What function $S(t)$ could satisfy this equation, such that its sum from 0 to infinity is $1/\mu$? If you remember calculus, you'll recall that the exponential function will do the job beautifully, as shown in Equation 4.3:

$$\int_0^\infty e^{-\mu t}dt \ = -\frac{e^{-\mu \times \infty} - e^{-\mu \times 0}}{\mu} = -\frac{0-1}{\mu} = \frac{1}{\mu}. \qquad \text{[Equation 4.3]}$$

So now we have a function to describe the probability that a Peep survives to time t, summarized in Equation 4.4:

$$S(t) = e^{-\mu t}. \qquad \text{[Equation 4.4]}$$

To recap, we have discovered two key learning points about rates of survival and durations of survival: the survival time in a state is the inverse of the rate of leaving a state; the probability of surviving in a state until time t can be expressed as an exponential rate of leaving the state.

AN INTRODUCTION TO QUEUING SYSTEMS

Many public health and healthcare services involve some supply, demand, and dropout. That is, some people are in need of a service (demand), we can provide some of them with that service they need (supply), but often people are caught waiting in line (queuing) and some of those people in line drop out of line before getting the service they need. For example, people might need a liver transplant, and there is some rate of new people being added to the organ transplant list. The number of people added per week is the rate of demand. The number of people on the waiting list at any given time is the length of the waiting line or the queue. The number of people getting a liver transplant per week is the rate of supply. But there are also, unfortunately, some people who never get a liver transplant and die while waiting for one; the rate of death on the list is the drop-out rate. This type of circumstance is diagrammed in Figure 4.3.

There are several key questions we might have if we are in charge of managing such a service. First, how can we most easily determine how many people are dropping out of the line because they aren't getting services in time? How many people might we prevent from dropping out if we were able to increase the number of people we could deliver services to by spending some additional budget dollars on the service? How much would demand need to decrease or supply need to increase for us to limit the waiting time for people we are serving to a reasonable level?

We can answer these questions by deriving two commonly used equations through the following example.

Suppose we are charged with operating a drug treatment program in the city of San Francisco. The City's Department of Public Health has a central treatment coordination center, at which anyone seeking drug treatment can sign up for service and health department workers will assist them to get drug rehabilitation.

Suppose that we know some data about this program based on information that is easy to collect, and that will help us answer some key questions about waiting lines and waiting times for this program. In particular, suppose that:

• An average of 100 people per month sign up for service (for drug rehabilitation).
• At the time of application, they are placed on a waiting list (queuing).
• New openings are available for people to enter the program at an average rate of 40 openings per month. In other words, 40 people are taken off the waiting list and placed into rehabilitation programs each month.
• Some people "drop off" the waiting list (they relapse to drug use).

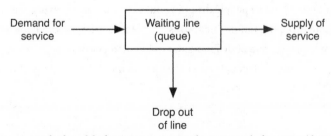

FIGURE 4.3 A standard model of queuing. Some people are in need of a service (demand), and we can provide some of them with that service they need (supply), but often people are caught waiting in line (queuing) and some of those people in line drop out of line before getting the service they need.

- People typically are able to stay off drugs and on the waiting list 2 months before they relapse. Therefore, the per-person rate of drop out is 1 person/2 months = 0.5/month, which can also be expressed as 0.5 months^{-1}.

For simplicity, let's suppose that whenever a new opening is available for a treatment program, the public health department attempts to contact the person on the waiting list; if the person has not dropped out of line (relapsed to drug use), they enroll into the drug rehabilitation program.

Given the information we have available, how many people do we anticipate will typically be waiting in line to receive rehabilitation services?

We can first solve the simplest, steady-state solution. The steady-state solution is the scenario in which the program has been operating for a long time without huge fluctuations in demand or supply from month to month (later, in a subsequent chapter, we'll solve for more complex situations that are in flux). Let L denote the steady-state number of people on the waiting list. To solve for the value of L, suppose that we characterize the problem with the following logic:

- We know the demand for services is 100 people per month.
- We know the supply of services is 40 openings per month (and hence 40 people can "receive service" and leave the waiting list for this reason each month).
- We know that the per person rate of dropping out of line is 0.5/month.
- Finally, we know that the complication we face is that people drop off the waiting list at a rate of 0.5 per person per month.

If the waiting list is at some steady-state value L, and people either leave the list by getting services or dropping out of line, then we know a critical piece of information: if 100 people enter the line per month, 100 people must leave the line per month. We know that 40 people fill openings in the center per month. Therefore, the other 60 people per month are drop-outs.

We can think of the 60 people dropping out of line in the following way: the number of people dropping out of line (60) is equal to the number of people in line (L) times the per-person rate of dropping out of line (0.5 per month).

Hence, we say that 100 people enter the line per month, and we have Equation 4.5:

$$60 = L \times 0.5. \qquad\qquad \text{[Equation 4.5]}$$

We can solve this expression to yield $L = 120$, which means that in our average steady-state circumstance, the line is 120 people long.

In calculating this solution, we have also derived a generalizable formula for calculating the steady-state number of people waiting in line at any given moment.

If we let the symbol δ (delta) denote the demand to enter the line per unit time, σ (sigma) denote the supply of services per unit time, and μ (mu) reflect the drop-out rate from the line, then we can produce a general equation reflecting the length L of the waiting line (or the "queue" in British-speak), shown in Equation 4.6:

$$L = \frac{(\delta - \sigma)}{\mu}. \qquad \text{[Equation 4.6]}$$

The length of a waiting line will typically equal the rate of demand minus the rate of supply, all divided by the rate of dropping out of line.

Suppose we have a question about the experience of people in line: how long do people typically have to wait to get service from our program, if they're folks who don't drop out but eventually get services?

We can solve for the waiting time of people who get service by first calculating the fraction of people who get into the program. The fraction who get into the program at steady state is proportional to the rate of service divided by the rate of demand, or σ/δ.

Looking at our Peeps example, the probability that a Peep (or person) survives until time t is given by Equation 4.4 and is the exponent of the negative rate of dropping-out times the time t.

The fraction of people who get into the program is the same as the probability of surviving the waiting time in line rather than dropping out of line. Hence, if the waiting time is W, we can write Equation 4.7:

$$\frac{\sigma}{\delta} = e^{-\mu W}. \qquad \text{[Equation 4.7]}$$

Hence, the time people typically spend waiting in line before getting surveyed can be expressed as Equation 4.8:

$$W = \left(\frac{1}{\mu}\right) ln\left(\frac{\delta}{\sigma}\right). \qquad \text{[Equation 4.8]}$$

The waiting time for service is the inverse of the drop-out rate, multiplied by an expression that depends on the ratio of the demand over supply.

In our example problem, the waiting time to obtain drug rehabilitation service is $(1/0.5)ln(100/40) = 1.8$ months. So the typical person who gets drug rehabilitation services would wait just under 2 months to receive services.

Having derived the two key equations—Equation 4.6 and Equation 4.8—to solve several problems, we can now estimate how much shorter our line would be if we add more service providers. Suppose, for example, that the San Francisco Department of Public Health added additional funds to increase the supply of drug rehabilitation facilities from 40 openings per month to 50 openings per month. How much shorter would the line be, and how much shorter would the waiting time be, until treatment?

Using Equation 4.6, we can solve that the waiting line would be $L = (100 - 50)/(0.5) = 100$ people long, rather than 120 people long. Using Equation 4.8, we can solve that the waiting time among people getting service would be $W = (1/0.5)ln(100/50) = 1.4$ months.

Critically, how many fewer people would drop out of line because they relapsed to drug use? That would typically be the number of people in line, L, multiplied by the rate of drop-out. So we would have $100 \times 0.5 = 50$ people dropping out per month, instead of the 60 people who dropped out of line when we only had 40 openings per month. Taking this information and combining it with cost data relating how much it costs the city in emergency room, jail, and crime costs for each active drug user, we could conduct a cost-effectiveness analysis as we did in Chapter 2—calculating whether the increased drug rehabilitation services are cost-effective from the perspective of the city government.

SOLVING QUEUING PROBLEMS WITH INADEQUATE INFORMATION

For many public health or healthcare problems, we lack sufficient detail about the exact rates of demand, supply, and drop-out rates, making it difficult to use Equations 4.6 and 4.8 to determine how long our consumers are waiting or how many fewer might drop out if we changed our supply of resources devoted to them.

Even with inadequate information, we can still use some common tricks to find the information we need and provide answers for key questions of interest.

Suppose we have the following problem:

During the cholera epidemic in Haiti in 2011, there was a shortage of a key antibiotic used to treat severe cholera cases. While most cholera cases are simply treated through administration of intravenous fluids, recent research suggested that, in severe cases, antibiotics would also help.

The organization Medicins Sans Frontieres (Doctors Without Borders) was running several field hospitals in Haiti and had to determine how many antibiotics to order. If they ordered too few antibiotics, patients would die. If they ordered too many, they wasted money that could have been spent on water purification equipment, intravenous tubing and needles, and other critical equipment and personnel costs.

When doctors at the hospital diagnosed people as having a case of severe cholera, they placed the patient on a waiting list to receive the antibiotic. On average, there were 39 people on the waiting list to receive the antibiotic. However, the actual number of people who received the antibiotic was about 7 per day due to inadequate supply. Not all those who entered the waiting list for the antibiotic received it (i.e., many people died), thus there was substantial "drop-out" from the antibiotic waiting list. For those who did receive antibiotics, the average waiting time was 3 days. Unfortunately, it was difficult to decipher any further information from the hospital because only these estimates were readily available given the antibiotic usage logs, waiting list, and interviews with patients who received treatment.

Based solely on this information, is it possible to estimate the true daily demand for antibiotics—that is, how many people actually needed antibiotics each day—so that the hospital manager could order the right amount?

To answer this question, we can first clarify what we know about this problem. We know that the typical length of the waiting line is $L = 39$ people, that the average rate of service is $\sigma = 7$ per day, and the duration people who get service are waiting in line is $W = 3$ days.

We can put the quantities we know into Equations 4.6 and 4.8. From Equation 4.6, we can see that:

$$L = \frac{(\delta - \sigma)}{\mu} = \frac{(\delta - 7)}{\mu} = 39.$$
[Equation 4.9]

Similarly, from Equation 4.8, we can see that:

$$W = \left(\frac{1}{\mu}\right) ln\left(\frac{\delta}{7}\right) = 3.$$
[Equation 4.10]

What we want to solve for is the value of daily demand, or δ. Unfortunately, neither equation can be solved on its own because we also lack information on the rate of drop-out from the list, μ.

A	B
Delta	10
Numerator	=B1-7
Denominator	=LN(B1/7)
Quotient	=B2/B3
Set equal to	13

FIGURE 4.4 Spreadsheet for solving the cholera queuing problem. We have created a spreadsheet in which the unknown variable δ is in cell B1, and set to an arbitrary value of 10 (we will later have Excel find its true value). We next set the numerator equal to the value of δ minus 7 by inserting the formula "=B1-7" into cell B2. We set the denominator equal to the value of $\ln(\delta/7)$ by inserting the formula "=LN(B1/7)" into cell B3. We calculate the quotient of the numerator and denominator in cell B4 by dividing cell B2 by cell B3—putting "=B2/B3" into cell B4. Finally, we put our target value for the quotient, the number 13, into cell B5.

Nevertheless, we can perform a mathematical trick by dividing Equation 4.9 by Equation 4.10. Doing so eliminates the unknown quantity μ:

$$\frac{\left[\dfrac{(\delta-7)}{\mu}=39\right]}{\left[\left(\dfrac{1}{\mu}\right)\ln\left(\dfrac{\delta}{7}\right)=3\right]} \text{ translates into } \frac{(\delta-7)}{\ln\left(\dfrac{\delta}{7}\right)}=13. \qquad \text{[Equation 4.11]}$$

Now we have one equation with just one unknown variable. The problem is that our unknown variable is not very easy to solve for, given the natural log in the denominator. We can use Excel to solve this problem for us by setting up the equation on our spreadsheet as shown in Figure 4.4.

As shown in Figure 4.4, we have created a spreadsheet in which the unknown variable δ is in cell B1 and set to an arbitrary value of 10 (we will later have Excel find its true value). We next set the numerator equal to the value of δ minus 7 by inserting the formula "=B1-7" into cell B2. We set the denominator equal to the value of $ln(\delta/7)$ by inserting the formula "=LN(B1/7)" into cell B3. We calculate the quotient of the numerator and denominator in cell B4 by dividing cell B2 by cell B3—putting "=B2/B3" into cell B4. Finally, we put our target value for the quotient, the number 13, into cell B5.

To enable Excel to find our solution for the value of δ, we go to "Tools" and then "Goal seek," which refers to a version of Solver without constraints. We want to set cell B4 to a value of 13 by changing cell B1. Figure 4.5 shows the appropriate input values for the Goal Seek dialog box.

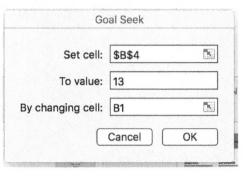

FIGURE 4.5 Solving the cholera queuing problem. To enable Excel to find our solution for the value of δ, we go to "Tools" and then "Goal seek", which refers to a version of Solver without constraints. We want to set cell B4 to a value of 13 by changing cell B1. The figure shows the appropriate input values for the Goal Seek dialog box.

Clicking "OK" and keeping the solution provides an estimated value of δ that is equal to 21.7, meaning that, on average, about 22 people are in need of antibiotics each day.

We can ask several additional questions based on our learning from this model. First, we can ask what fraction of people in need of antibiotics actually receives them given the current rates of service and demand?

We can reason that the fraction of those needing antibiotics who actually receive them is the rate of service (σ) divided by the rate of demand (δ), or $7/22 = 0.32$. In other words, only about one-third of people who need antibiotic treatment are receiving it.

Another question is: if all people enter into the waiting line immediately upon getting sick and drop out of the waiting line because they are dying, what's the typical survival time for a person with severe cholera?

The survival time for a person with a disease is the inverse of the mortality rate (Equation 4.1). Here, the mortality rate is the same as the rate of dropping out of line, μ. Hence, to calculate the survival time, we have to calculate the value of $1/\mu$. We can use either Equation 4.6 or Equation 4.8 to get our estimate.

From Equation 4.6, we have:

$$1/\mu = L/(\delta - \sigma) = 39/(22 - 7) = 2.6 \text{ days.} \qquad \text{[Equation 4.12]}$$

Similarly, from Equation 4.8, we have:

$$1/\mu = W/ln(\delta/\sigma) = 3/(ln(22/7)) = 2.6 \text{ days.} \qquad \text{[Equation 4.13]}$$

Either way, we see that the average person survives a very short period of under 3 days when afflicted with severe cholera.

5

MODELING HEALTH INTERVENTIONS

In this chapter, we will examine one of the most common and useful ways to understand complex public health and healthcare interventions: the *Markov model*. A Markov model is a representation of health or disease that expands well beyond the simple queuing model we created in Chapter 4. In that chapter, we studied just one "state"—a waiting line—and examined how changes to the rates of flow in and out of that state (rates of demand, putting people into the waiting line; rates of service or drop-out, taking people out of the waiting line) affected the length of the line and the duration people waited in line. In this chapter, we will use Markov models to expand our analysis to many more possible states, such as multiple stages of disease, to identify how effective or cost-effective our public health and healthcare programs might be. Markov models are highly flexible and allow for an infinite variety of diseases or interventions to be simulated and understood, which is why they are among the most popular tools for public health and healthcare research.

PRINCIPLES OF MARKOV MODELING: AN EXAMPLE FROM THE COCAINE EPIDEMIC

In the 1980s, an epidemic of cocaine drug abuse debilitated many cities across the United States. People who used the drug flooded emergency rooms with complications of drug use, such as heart problems and complications of pregnancy. Indebtedness and crime related to cocaine abuse devastated many of the country's poorest neighborhoods.

In Los Angeles, a city health commission was formed to investigate strategies to mitigate the cocaine epidemic. The commission set about the task of addressing the epidemic by trying to understand just how bad the problem really was. But typical strategies they relied on to assess the burden of cocaine abuse in the community were not working. At first, they tried a household survey. Few people would open their front door for a surveyor from the health department, and even fewer would admit to abusing cocaine, even if the survey was anonymous.

The health department officials searched for an alternative approach to understand how common the epidemic was. They sought to "back-calculate" the typical incidence and prevalence rates of the disease from the limited information they were able to obtain from Drug Enforcement Administration (DEA) databases and interviews with medical experts at local hospitals who treated people for complications of cocaine abuse. There were a few key pieces of information they were able to deduce from these records alone.

First, they were able to confirm that only a small portion of the population actually ended up using cocaine at all. Local drug dealers usually sold to a limited number of clients who shared the drug among their social networks. On average, they estimated that, in their city, people who never used cocaine had only a 0.5% probability per month of starting to use it and would use it only rarely. Medical experts also estimated that rare users would quit by the next month 15% of the time and only become routine (daily) users of cocaine over the next month about 2.4% of the time. Among the routine, daily users of cocaine, many people would remain heavy cocaine users; few would lapse back into rare use (at a rate of about 4% per month), while another 2% per month would quit altogether and become nonusers of cocaine again. No one was believed to transition directly from nonuse to routine daily use, and the risk of death from cocaine use was actually found to be exceedingly rare, effectively less than 0.1% per month, despite much public hype about the drug's dangers.

The health commission decided that this information could help them construct a fundamental understanding of cocaine use in their city. They created a diagram for how cocaine was being used and how many people ended up staying routine users who might benefit from further drug addiction treatment.

To make use of this information, the health commission constructed a Markov model, also known as a Markov chain, which diagrams a complex sequence of possible outcomes as a chain of possible "health states" that people can occupy. A Markov model can be conceptualized as a series of lily pads on which a frog is jumping. The pads are different states of health or disease. The frog jumping across the pads is like a person going between these states of health or disease. The key features of a Markov model are a *state diagram*, which clearly designates the possible health states that can be occupied as a sequence of connected circles, and *state transitions*, or arrows that identify the probability of moving from one state to another.

Figure 5.1 illustrates a state diagram for the Los Angeles cocaine epidemic.

In this state diagram, we can see that there are three possible states of cocaine use: being a nonuser of cocaine, being a rare user of cocaine, or being a routine user of cocaine. Given the very low risk of death, the department did not include death in their Markov model, although later we will see how it could easily be added to the model. The three health states are connected by state transition probabilities

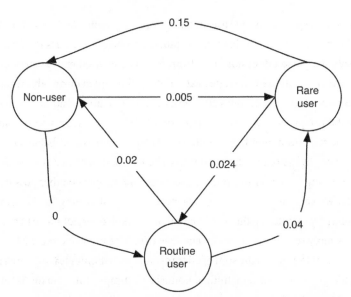

FIGURE 5.1 State diagram for the Markov model of Los Angeles's cocaine epidemic. There are three possible states of cocaine use: being a non-user of cocaine, being a rare user of cocaine, or being a routine user of cocaine. Given the very low risk of death, death is not included in the Markov model. The three health states are connected by state transition probabilities that describe how likely it is for a person to transition from one state to the other. There is a probability of 0.005 per month of a nonuser becoming a rare user of cocaine, a probability of 0.15 per month of a light user becoming a nonuser, a probability of 0.024 per month of the rare user becoming a routine user, a probability of 0.04 per month of a heavy user becoming a rare user, and a probability of 0.02 of per month heavy user becoming a non-user. There is also a zero probability of going from non-user to routine user.

that describe how likely it is for a person to transition from one state to the other. It is important to ensure that we use the same units of time across all possible transitions between one state and another; in this case, all state transition probabilities are in monthly units, also known as monthly *time steps*. Markov models are said to be *irreducible* if it is possible to get to any state from any other state, as in this example.

We know there is a probability of 0.005 per month of a nonuser becoming a rare user of cocaine, a probability of 0.15 per month of a light user becoming a nonuser, a probability of 0.024 per month of the rare user becoming a routine user, a probability of 0.04 per month of a heavy user becoming a rare user, and a probability of 0.02 of per month heavy user becoming a nonuser. There is also a zero probability of going from nonuser to routine user. These probabilities are illustrated in Figure 5.1.

Our Markov model can help us translate our information about the nature of cocaine use to estimate the incidence or prevalence of cocaine use in Los Angeles and determine how many people might need substance abuse treatment for routine cocaine use. To calculate these estimates using our Markov model, we need to complete our state diagram by adding all possible transition probabilities between states in our diagram. To do so, we can reason that our state diagram captures all possible states of health with respect to cocaine use. In other words, a person who lives in Los Angeles cannot be in a state of health that is not captured by one of the circles in our diagram. As a result, if a person does not move from one state to another, we can reason that they are remaining in the same state next month as they are in during this month (i.e., a nonuser who does not become a cocaine user must remain a nonuser). Hence, there is a probability equal to 1 of either leaving a state to come to another state or remaining in the same state from month to month. For example, there is a probability of 1 that a person either stays a nonuser, transitions from being a nonuser to a rare user, or transitions from being a nonuser to a routine user (there are simply no other possibilities).

Hence, we can calculate *self-loops*, or probabilities of staying in the same state each month, by calculating the probability that a person does not move to a different state but simply remains in their current state from one month to the next. The self-loops are equal to 1 minus the sum of all transition probabilities leaving a given state. Hence, the probability of remaining a nonuser next month if a person is already a nonuser is equal to 1 minus the probability of transitioning from a nonuser to a rare user minus the probability of transitioning from a nonuser to a routine user, or $1 - 0.005 - 0 = 0.995$. Similarly, the probability of remaining a rare user next month if a person is already a rare user is equal to 1 minus the probability of transitioning from a rare user to a nonuser minus the probability of transitioning from a rare user to a routine user, or $1 - 0.15 - 0.024 = 0.826$. Finally, the probability of remaining a routine user next month if a person is already a routine user is equal to 1 minus the probability of transitioning from a routine user to a nonuser minus the probability of transitioning from a routine user to a rare user, or $1 - 0.02 - 0.04 = 0.94$. These self-loop transition probabilities are labeled as curved arrows on Figure 5.2, which provides a complete state diagram for our Markov model.

We can check that we haven't made a mistake in our model by adding all of the transition probabilities that leave a given state, including self-loop transition probabilities; the sum of all probabilities must add to 1 since people cannot disappear from our diagram.

Now that we have established the state diagram for our Markov model, we can use the model to answer several critical questions about the Los Angeles cocaine epidemic. To start with, we can ask, in a population of about 4 million people, how many people would we expect to be cocaine users given the data we have available?

At first, this question may seem impossible to answer since we only have limited information about the probabilities that any individual might transition between different levels of cocaine use, not information about the overall epidemic in the population of Los Angeles. But one of the key strengths of a Markov model is its ability to translate data from the level of the individual to the level of the population. To see this advantage of Markov modeling, we can translate our state diagram

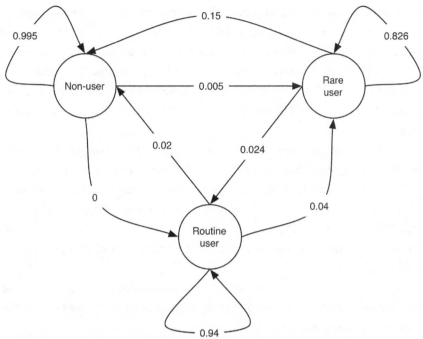

FIGURE 5.2 **State diagram for the Markov model of Los Angeles's cocaine epidemic, after including self-loops, or probabilities of staying in the same state each month. The self-loops are equal to 1 minus the sum of all transition probabilities leaving a given state. Hence, the probability of remaining a non-user next month if a person is already a non-user is equal to 1 – the probability of transitioning from a non-user to a rare user minus the probability of transitioning from a non-user to a routine user, or 1 – 0.005 – 0 = 0.995. Similarly, the probability of remaining a rare user next month if a person is already a rare user is equal to 1 – the probability of transitioning from a rare user to a non-user minus the probability of transitioning from a rare user to a routine user, or 1 – 0.15 – 0.024 = 0.826. Finally, the probability of remaining a routine user next month if a person is already a routine user is equal to 1 – the probability of transitioning from a routine user to a non-user minus the probability of transitioning from a routine user to a rare user, or 1 – 0.02 – 0.04 = 0.94.**

into a series of equations. Let $p_{non}(t)$, $p_{rare}(t)$, and $p_{routine}(t)$ refer to the probabilities that a person is a nonuser, rare user, or routine user in any given month t. If we read our state diagram as a description of the probability that a person shifts from one state to another with each passing month, then we can write Equations 5.1 through 5.4:

$$p_{non}(t+1) = 0.995 p_{non}(t) + 0.15 p_{rare}(t) + 0.02 p_{routine}(t) \qquad \text{[Equation 5.1]}$$

$$p_{rare}(t+1) = 0.005 p_{non}(t) + 0.826 p_{rare}(t) + 0.04 p_{routine}(t) \qquad \text{[Equation 5.2]}$$

$$p_{routine}(t+1) = 0 p_{non}(t) + 0.024 p_{rare}(t) + 0.94 p_{routine}(t) \qquad \text{[Equation 5.3]}$$

$$p_{non}(t) + p_{rare}(t) + p_{routine}(t) = 1. \qquad \text{[Equation 5.4]}$$

Equation 5.1 states that the probability of being a nonuser in month $t + 1$ is the probability of being a nonuser in month t times 0.995, plus the probability of being a rare user in month t times 0.15, plus the probability of being a routine user in month t times 0.02. In other words, the probability of being a nonuser in month $t + 1$ is the probability of moving over from any state to the nonuser state over the course of 1 month, including the probability of staying a nonuser from month t to month $t + 1$.

Similarly, we can see from Figure 5.2 that Equation 5.2 is the sum of all probabilities that move a person from any state to the rare user state. Finally, Equation 5.3 is the sum of all probabilities that move a person from any state to a routine user state.

The final equation, Equation 5.4, tells us that people cannot magically disappear from our state diagram. A person who is alive in Los Angeles must be a nonuser, rare user, or routine user of cocaine, and, therefore, the sum of all three probabilities must be equal to 1.

Equations 5.1 through 5.4 are commonly termed *difference equations* because they express the difference in the probability of being in a state at time $t + 1$ and the probability of being in a state at time t.

How do we use these equations to help us understand the cocaine epidemic? The easiest strategy to utilize these equations is to first solve for the probability of being in each state under a *steady-state situation*, that is, over the long-term after much time has passed and the probability of being in each state doesn't vary much over time. After we perform an algebraic solution to the problem, we will later illustrate that Markov models typically have a long-term *stationary distribution*, or a long-term steady state probability for an individual to be in any one of the given states. For now, we can take it on faith that such a long-term probability exists, and later we will demonstrate its existence more rigorously.

Over the long term, we can reason that the probability of being in any given state is so stable that it does not change from one time step to another. Hence, we no longer need to think of transitions from time t to time $t + 1$ and can rewrite Equations 5.1 and 5.4 as their steady-state versions, Equations 5.5 through 5.8:

$$P_{non} = 0.995 p_{non} + 0.15 p_{rare} + 0.02 p_{routine} \qquad \text{[Equation 5.5]}$$

$$P_{rare} = 0.005 p_{non} + 0.826 p_{rare} + 0.04 p_{routine} \qquad \text{[Equation 5.6]}$$

$$P_{routine} = 0 p_{non} + 0.024 p_{rare} + 0.94 p_{routine} \qquad \text{[Equation 5.7]}$$

$$P_{non} + P_{rare} + P_{routine} = 1. \qquad \text{[Equation 5.8]}$$

Equations 5.5 through 5.8 assume that, over the long run, the epidemic of cocaine use will stabilize such that the probability of being a nonuser will not vary dramatically from month to month, nor will the probability of being a rare user or the probability of being a routine user.

Because Equations 5.5 through 5.8 provide us with three unknown terms (p_{non}, p_{rare}, and $p_{routine}$) and four equations, we can solve them algebraically. We can first solve for p_{non} in terms of p_{rare} and $p_{routine}$ using Equation 5.5, then substitute the expression for p_{non} into Equation 5.6 to solve for p_{rare} in terms of $p_{routine}$, and finally substitute the expression for p_{rare} into Equation 5.7 or Equation 5.8 to solve for the numerical value of $p_{routine}$ at steady state. We can then compute the other two numerical probabilities using our equations, which solve to yield $p_{non} = 0.958$, $p_{rare} = 0.030$, and $p_{routine} = 0.012$. In other words, over the long-term, we would expect that most people (95.7%) are nonusers of cocaine, few people (3.1%) are rare users, and even fewer (1.2%) are routine users of cocaine.

Those students who recall linear algebra can also choose to express Equations 5.5 through 5.8 as a series of matrices, as shown in Equation 5.9, which can be solved with matrix multiplication to obtain the same solution:

$$
\begin{bmatrix}
0.995 & 0.15 & 0.02 \\
0.005 & 0.826 & 0.04 \\
0 & 0.024 & 0.94
\end{bmatrix}
\begin{bmatrix}
p_{non} \\
p_{rare} \\
p_{routine}
\end{bmatrix}
=
\begin{bmatrix}
p_{non} \\
p_{rare} \\
p_{routine}
\end{bmatrix}.
\qquad \text{[Equation 5.9]}
$$

The three-by-three matrix of transition probabilities is commonly referred to as a *transition matrix*.

Both strategies for solving the problem are someone tedious so, in the next section, we reveal a strategy to solve for the probabilities using Excel rather than solving the problem by hand. No matter which way we solve the problem, we should obtain the same steady-state solution.

Using our solution to the steady-state equations, we can solve our problem regarding how many people we expect to be cocaine users in Los Angeles. Over the long-term, we anticipate that the prevalence of cocaine use will be the number of people in the population (about 4 million for Los Angeles) multiplied by the probability that each person will be using cocaine (both the probability of rare use and the probability of routine use), as expressed in Equation 5.10:

$$
4{,}000{,}000 \times \left(p_{rare} + p_{routine}\right) = 4{,}000{,}000 \times \left(0.030 + 0.012\right) = 168{,}000.
$$
$$
\text{[Equation 5.10]}
$$

In other words, about 168,000 people would be expected to be using cocaine either rarely or routinely in Los Angeles over the long term.

In the next section, we will learn how to program our model into Excel to solve for the probability of being in any state before the long-term steady-state, such as during the early epidemic years when the use of cocaine may be acutely increasing with every passing month.

Before we implement the model in Excel, we can still answer several important questions by hand based on our model equations. We can not only identify the likely *prevalence* of disease, but also identify estimates of the *incidence* of new disease, meaning how many people start becoming users of cocaine from the nonuse state.

What would be the typical incidence rate of becoming a rare user if starting out as a nonuser? The probability per month of becoming a rare user from a nonuser is 0.5% or 0.005 per month. The absolute number of people who are nonusers in a given month is $p_{non} = 0.958$. Hence, the incidence in the population per month of becoming a rare user of cocaine would be expressed by Equation 5.11:

$$4{,}000{,}000 \times p_{non} \times 0.005 = 4{,}000{,}000 \times 0.958 \times 0.005 = 19{,}160. \qquad \text{[Equation 5.11]}$$

Hence, we expect just over 19,000 people per month become rare users of cocaine from the nonuser state. Note that this calculation is not isolating people who have never used cocaine before, but rather is calculating the incidence rate of rare cocaine use after including all people who are currently in the nonusing state. A particular individual might have used cocaine in the past but has returned to the nonuser state, and, if they relapse to rare cocaine use, would be included in our incident rate calculation.

The calculation of incidence reveals an important property of Markov models: the so-called Markov assumption, or *memoryless* property. A Markov model does not capture a person's prior history when estimating the person's probability of transitioning from one state to another. A person who has never used cocaine before is given the same probability of becoming a rare user as someone who has previously recovered from routine cocaine use. This is unrealistic, but the fact that the Markov model lacks memory for a person's prior history makes the mathematics governing the model more convenient. Sometimes, modelers will add more states to a Markov model to differentiate people with a prior history of a condition from people without such a history, although this adds more states and more equations to a model, making it more complex. In a Chapter 8, we will introduce microsimulation modeling methods, which can resolve this problem. For now, let us use the simplest model for illustrative purposes.

The simple Markov model we have created can assist us to plan an intervention to help reduce the cocaine epidemic. Suppose a drug treatment program was designed to help people who are routine users of cocaine. How many people should we plan to serve initially in our program?

If we are isolating our treatment to only routine cocaine users, then we would anticipate that the demand for the program would isolate the number of people in our population (about 4 million for Los Angeles) multiplied by the probability that each person will be using cocaine routinely, as expressed in Equation 5.12:

$$4,000,000 \times p_{routine} = 4,000,000 \times 0.012 = 48,000. \qquad \text{[Equation 5.12]}$$

We would plan to treat about 48,000 people for our initial pool of eligible routine cocaine users. What would be the long-term decline in routine use given our program? Suppose our program increases the rate at which routine users become nonusers from the current probability of 2% or 0.02 per month to twice the current rate, or 4% or 0.04 per month. We can envision that this increased probability of recovering from cocaine use would reduce the self-loop probability of staying a routine user from 0.94 to 0.92 per month (so that the total probability of staying a routine user or moving to either nonuser or rare use still sums to a value of 1, as is required, since people cannot move out of one of the three states or appear from nowhere).

We can depict the change in our model following this intervention by rewriting Equations 5.5 through 5.8 as Equations 5.13 through 5.16:

$$p_{non} = 0.995 p_{non} + 0.15 p_{rare} + \mathbf{0.04p_{routine}} \qquad \text{[Equation 5.13]}$$

$$p_{rare} = 0.005 p_{non} + 0.826 p_{rare} + 0.04 p_{routine} \qquad \text{[Equation 5.14]}$$

$$p_{routine} = 0 p_{non} + 0.024 p_{rare} + \mathbf{0.92p_{routine}} \qquad \text{[Equation 5.15]}.$$

$$p_{non} + p_{rare} + p_{routine} = 1. \qquad \text{[Equation 5.16]}$$

The two changes capturing the impact of our intervention are reflected in bold: a change from $0.02 p_{routine}$ to $0.04 p_{routine}$ in Equation 5.13, and a change from $0.94 p_{routine}$ to $0.92 p_{routine}$ in Equation 5.15.

If we were to solve these equations, we would see a subtle change in the solution for the stationary distribution transition probabilities. Before our drug treatment intervention, Equations 5.5 through 5.8 solved to yield $p_{non} = 0.958$, $p_{rare} = 0.030$, and $p_{routine} = 0.012$. After our drug treatment intervention, Equations 5.13 through 5.16 solved to yield $p_{non} = 0.961$, $p_{rare} = 0.030$, and $p_{routine} = 0.009$. Hence, the probability of being a routine user of cocaine has, because of our intervention, been reduced from 0.012 to 0.009. Overall, the prevalence of routine cocaine use in the Los Angeles population would be expected to lower from 48,000 before our intervention to:

$$4,000,000 \times p_{routine} = 4,000,000 \times 0.009 = 36,000. \qquad \text{[Equation 5.17]}$$

We expect that our intervention would help lower the prevalence of routine cocaine use by 48,000 − 36,000 = 12,000 people in the city of Los Angeles.

In addition to calculating the lower *prevalence* of cocaine use, we might also ask whether our intervention has indirect benefits in terms of altering the *incidence* of cocaine use. The absolute number of people who are nonusers in a given month is now p_{non} = 0.961 after the intervention. Hence, the incidence in the population per month of becoming a rare user of cocaine would be expressed by Equation 5.18:

$$4,000,000 \times p_{non} \times 0.005 = 4,000,000 \times 0.961 \times 0.005 = 19,220. \qquad \text{[Equation 5.18]}$$

While our previous incidence per month was 19,160, we now have a higher incidence of rare cocaine use of 19,220 because the overall population of nonusers is now higher (more routine users have quit), but the probability of becoming a rare user from a nonuser has not changed. This doesn't indicate that our intervention is "bad thing" because we have still lowered the overall probability of being a routine user. The result simply highlights that the outcomes of Markov models can be complex, and we should look carefully at how indirect effects between states can lead to surprising conclusions.

Is our intervention cost-effective? In the next section, we will program our model into Excel in order to estimate the cost-effectiveness of the intervention and realize the potential of using a Markov model to estimate the population-level benefits of a health intervention.

BEYOND STEADY-STATE SOLUTIONS: IMPLEMENTATION IN EXCEL

To find the steady-state stationary distribution probabilities of a Markov model more easily, it's possible to program the model into Excel, saving us the trouble of doing algebra or matrix multiplication by hand. Programming the model into Excel also allows us to estimate the prevalence and incidence of disease in non–steady-state conditions and estimate the cost-effectiveness of our intervention more easily.

To program the model in Excel, we first create a standard format for inputting Markov model matrices into a spreadsheet. The spreadsheet that accompanies the chapter in this book online (https://github.com/sanjaybasu/modelinghealthsystems/)

provides a template corresponding to our cocaine example, which is illustrated in Figure 5.3 and can be easily expanded to other Markov models.

On the left-hand side of the spreadsheet shown in Figure 5.3 is our transition matrix, just as it appears in Equation 5.9. The matrix rows correspond to the transition probabilities of *entering into* a given state, and the matrix columns correspond to the transition probabilities of *coming from* a given state. For example, row 2 column 1 is the transition probability 0.005, which is the probability of entering into the rare user state from the nonuser state.

On the right-hand side of the spreadsheet shown in Figure 5.3 is the model implementation space. We have four columns that we create in this space. First, we create a column for each time step of our simulation. In this case, we are counting time in months, and so each time step corresponds to a new month. To quickly fill in this row, we can simply type in the value "1" in the first row of the time column, which appears in cell G2. Below cell G2, in cell G3, we can type the formula "=G2+1," which tells Excel to calculate 1 plus the value of cell G2 into cell G3. We can then left-click on the corner of cell G3 and drag our mouse down column G to fill in the rest of the column by having Excel fill in the months sequentially. In our example, we will simulate 120 months (10 years) of the epidemic, so we can drag through row 121 and Excel should automatically fill in the month numbers from 2 through 120.

Next, we have the three columns that correspond to our three states of cocaine use. In cells H2, I2, and J2, we have arbitrarily put in "1" as the starting value for the probability of being a nonuser in month 1 and "0" as the probability of being a rare user or routine user in month 1, under the assumption that, before the cocaine epidemic begins, no one is yet using cocaine (these are referred to as the *initial conditions* of the model specification). The next row is the most complex and important to understand: it is the row in which we insert our equations. In cell H3, we insert Equation 5.1, the equation indicating the probability of being a nonuser in month 2, given the probabilities of being a nonuser, rare user, or routine user in month 1. In

	A	B	C	D	E	F	G	H	I	J
1	Transition matrix			Coming from:			Time (month)	P(non)	P(rare)	P(routine)
2			nonuser	rare user	routine user		1	1	0	0
3		nonuser	0.995	0.15	0.02		=G2+1	=C$3*H2+D$3*I2+E$3*J2	=C$4*H2+D$4*I2+E$4*J2	=C$5*H2+D$5*I2+E$5*J2
4	Entering into:	rare user	0.005	0.826	0.04					
5		routine user	0	0.024	0.94					

FIGURE 5.3 Implementation of the Markov model of Los Angeles's cocaine epidemic in Excel. On the left-hand side of the spreadsheet shown in Figure 5.3 is our transition matrix, just as it appears in Equation 5.9. The matrix rows correspond to the transition probabilities of *entering into* a given state, and the matrix columns correspond to the transition probabilities of *coming from* a given state. On the right-hand side of the spreadsheet shown in Figure 5.3 is the model implementation space. We have four columns that we create in this space. First, we create a column for each time step of our simulation. Next, we have the three columns that correspond to our three states of cocaine use. The next row is the row in which we insert our equations. In cell H3, we insert Equation 5.1; in cell I3 we insert Equation 5.2; and in cell J3 we insert Equation 5.3.

Excel language, we insert the expression "=C$3*H2+D$3*I2+E$3*J2" into cell H3. This expression tells Excel to look into cell C3 (the transition matrix) to give us the value 0.995 of a nonuser staying a nonuser, and multiply it by cell H2, the probability of being a nonuser in month 1; then Excel should add this product to the product of cell D3 (the probability 0.15 of moving from rare-user to nonuser) and multiply it by cell I2 (the probability of being a rare user in month 1); finally, Excel should add to the expression the product of cell E2 (the probability 0.02 of moving from routine user to nonuser) and multiply it by cell J2 (the probability of being a routine user in month 1). The reason we add a dollar sign in front of the 3's in the expression is that we will later click and drag this expression down to calculate its value across all time points. When doing so, we want Excel to always refer to the correct row of the transition matrix. If we don't have dollar signs in front of the numbers, then Excel will adjust the formula to correspond to the next number in a sequence; for example, H2 will become H3 when we copy the formula to the next row. The dollar signs prevent Excel from changing the row of the transition matrix, ensuring we have the correct value for the probability of transitioning from one state to another.

Similarly, in cell I3, we insert Equation 5.2, the equation indicating the probability of being a rare user in month 2, given the probabilities of being a nonuser, rare user, or routine user in month 1. In Excel language, we insert the expression "=C$4*H2+D$4*I2+E$4*J2" into cell I3.

Finally, in cell J3, we insert Equation 5.3, the equation indicating the probability of being a routine user in month 2, given the probabilities of being a nonuser, rare user, or routine user in month 1. In Excel language, we insert the expression "=C$5*H2+D$5*I2+E$5*J2" into cell J3.

We should now have a spreadsheet that looks like Figure 5.3.

To complete our model, we now have to allow Excel to calculate the Markov model for all subsequent months over our chosen *time horizon*, or the duration of the model that we wish to simulate. In this case, we want to simulate a time horizon of 10 years, or 120 month. Hence, we should highlight cells G3 through J3 and left-click and drag them down through row 121. Doing so will allow Excel to automatically calculate the probabilities of being in each state for each subsequent month of the simulation, as shown in Figure 5.4.

The spreadsheet will reveal that a steady-state stationary distribution is achieved among all three states of the model. In particular, if we scroll down to month 120, we see that the probabilities of being in each state correspond to the probabilities we calculated by hand of $p_{non} = 0.958$, $p_{rare} = 0.030$, and $p_{routine} = 0.012$. By implementing the model in Excel, we have saved ourselves the pain of having to calculate the probabilities using algebra and should expect to see the stationary distribution estimates after a sufficiently long period of time steps have passed in the Excel model.

G	H	I	J
Time (month)	P(non)	P(rare)	P(routine)
1	1	0	0
2	0.995	0.005	0
3	0.990775	0.009105	0.00012
4	0.98718928	0.01247941	0.00033132
5	0.98413187	0.01525719	0.00061095
6	0.981512	0.01754753	0.00094046
7	0.97925538	0.01943944	0.00130518
8	0.97730113	0.02100546	0.00169341
9	0.97559931	0.02230475	0.00209594
10	0.97410894	0.02338556	0.0025055
11	0.97279634	0.02428724	0.00291642
12	0.97163377	0.0250419	0.00332433
13	0.97059838	0.02567575	0.00372587
14	0.96967127	0.0262102	0.00411854
15	0.96883681	0.02666272	0.00450047
16	0.96808204	0.02704761	0.00487035
17	0.96739618	0.02737655	0.00522727
18	0.96677023	0.0276591	0.00557067
19	0.96619665	0.0279031	0.00590025
20	0.96566914	0.02811495	0.00621591
21	0.96518236	0.02829993	0.00651771
22	0.96473179	0.02846236	0.00680585
23	0.9643136	0.02860581	0.00708059
24	0.96392452	0.02873319	0.0073423
25	0.96356172	0.02884693	0.00759136
26	0.96322277	0.02894902	0.0078282
27	0.96290558	0.02904114	0.00805329
28	0.96260829	0.02912464	0.00826708
29	0.96232928	0.02920068	0.00847004
30	0.96206714	0.02927021	0.00866266
31	0.96182059	0.02933403	0.00884538

FIGURE 5.4 Implementation of the Markov model of Los Angeles's cocaine epidemic in Excel. The spreadsheet will reveal that a steady-state stationary distribution is achieved among all three states of the model.

By highlighting the four columns and clicking the "Insert" menu item, then clicking "Chart" and "X Y (Scatter)" chart option, we can plot the overall course of the cocaine epidemic in Los Angeles across the simulated months. As shown in Figure 5.5, the chart reveals a gradual increase from zero cocaine use to the steady-state stationary prevalence rates of use. Hence, the Excel version of the model also permits us to easily identify what the prevalence of cocaine use might be in early parts of the epidemic, not just in the steady-state long-term case. As shown, if we scroll down to month 12 of our model spreadsheet, we would expect only about 2.5% cocaine use in the first year of the epidemic, as compared to the long-term prevalence of more than 3.1% cocaine use (including both rare and routine use).

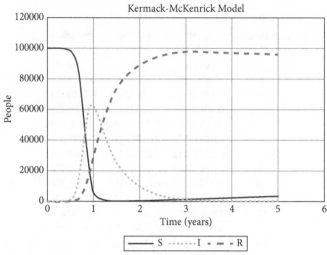

FIGURE 5.5 Results of the Markov model of Los Angeles's cocaine epidemic. Note a gradual increase from zero cocaine use to a steady-state stationary prevalence of use.

By inserting our model into Excel, we have also gained two key advantages over solving the model by hand: (1) we have gained the ability to quickly visualize how the epidemic would be expected to change once the initial conditions of the model change or if the transition matrix changes (such as by introducing a new public health intervention), and (2) we have gained the ability to leverage the model for comparative effectiveness analysis (comparing different interventions) and cost-effectiveness analysis (estimating the incremental cost-effectiveness of introducing a new program).

Let us illustrate each of these two functionalities in turn. First, we can use our new model to quickly visualize how the epidemic would be expected to change once the initial conditions of the model change or if the transition matrix changes (such as by introducing a new public health intervention). We can easily see how the epidemic might change given different initial conditions by changing cells H2 through J2. Suppose we changed the values to indicate that, in month 1 of the model, there is already a 5% chance of being a rare user of cocaine and a 1% chance of being a routine user (leaving a 94% chance of being a nonuser). Hence, cells H2 through J2 would be 0.94, 0.05, and 0.01. If we insert these values into cells H2 through J2, we see that the epidemic takes on an initially different shape but the transition matrix, not the initial conditions, dictate the long-term steady-state stationary distribution of probabilities. While the probabilities of being a cocaine user at month 12 are higher (about 3.3%), the long-term steady-state stationary probabilities remain the same (at 3.1%, including both rare and routine use).

Next, suppose we start the epidemic back at the initial condition values of $p_{non} = 1$, $p_{rare} = 0$, and $p_{routine} = 0$. What happens if we change the transition matrix by including our drug treatment program, which increases the rate at which routine users become nonusers from the current probability of 2% or 0.02 per month to twice the current rate, or 4% or 0.04 per month? We can create a copy of our model to illustrate what would happen with the drug treatment in place by right-clicking on the "Sheet1" tab at the bottom and selecting "Move or Copy," then selecting "(move to end)" and checking the "create a copy" box. The sequence of steps will produce a new copy of our model in a second sheet or tab. Suppose in this new sheet that we change the transition matrix to correspond to the postintervention transition matrix, reflected in Equations 5.13 through 5.16. We change the top right cell in our transition matrix (cell E3) from 0.02 to 0.04, and we change the bottom right cell (cell E5) from 0.94 to 0.92. Note that the sum of each column should still equal 1, reflecting that a person must be in one of the three states of our model at all times.

Once we change the transition matrix, we can see that the new steady-state stationary probabilities values are $p_{non} = 0.961$, $p_{rare} = 0.030$, and $p_{routine} = 0.009$, just as we calculated earlier. So we have lowered the probability of being a routine user from 0.012 to 0.009 through our program.

Suppose we now wish to utilize our model to perform comparative effectiveness analysis (comparing different interventions) or cost-effectiveness analysis (estimating the incremental cost-effectiveness of introducing a new program). In particular, suppose we wish to compare the effectiveness of this intervention, which treats routine drug users, with an alternative intervention that aims to reduce the probability of becoming a rare user under the logic that preventing rare use will prevent future routine use and that prevention is better than treatment. Figure 5.6 illustrates the comparison.

On the left hand side of Figure 5.6 is the intervention we are currently simulating: the introduction of a treatment program for routine users. The figure illustrates how we conceptualize the increase in the rate of quitting among routine users who become nonusers because of the intervention. On the right hand side of Figure 5.6 is the alternative intervention proposed: the introduction of a prevention program to avert rare use. The figure illustrates how we envision the rate of rare use being cut in half by the program.

To simulate the prevention program, we can create a third spreadsheet in our Excel file by right-clicking on the "Sheet1" tab at the bottom and selecting "Move or Copy" then selecting "(move to end)" and checking the "create a copy" box. We then insert the transition matrix that corresponds to our prevention intervention, which—reading from Figure 5.6—should have the transition matrix shown in Equation 5.19, where bold text indicates the changes from the preintervention simulation of Equation 5.9 (a cut in half of the rate of transition

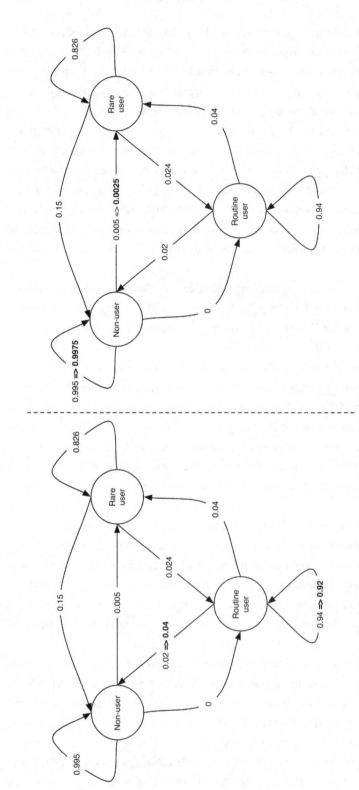

FIGURE 5.6 Using Markov models to compare the effectiveness of a prevention and a treatment intervention for cocaine use. On the left hand side is the introduction of a treatment program for routine users. On the right hand side is the introduction of a prevention program to avert rare use.

from nonuse to rare use and a corresponding increase in the rate of staying a nonuser):

$$
\begin{bmatrix} 0.9975 & 0.15 & 0.02 \\ 0.0025 & 0.826 & 0.04 \\ 0 & 0.024 & 0.94 \end{bmatrix}
\begin{bmatrix} p_{non} \\ p_{rare} \\ p_{routine} \end{bmatrix}
=
\begin{bmatrix} p_{non} \\ p_{rare} \\ p_{routine} \end{bmatrix}.
\qquad \text{[Equation 5.19]}
$$

If we type the transition matrix in correctly, we should obtain steady-state station-ary probability values of p_{non} = 0.978, p_{rare} = 0.015, and $p_{routine}$ = 0.006. Hence, we can immediately identify that the prevention program produces a lower rate of both rare and routine cocaine use than the treatment program; the prevention program produces an overall 1.5% + 0.6% = 2.1% prevalence of cocaine, versus a 3.0% + 0.9% = 3.9% prevalence of cocaine from the treatment program.

Now suppose we want to conduct a cost-effectiveness analysis to compare the incre-mental cost-effectiveness of the treatment program to the baseline (no intervention) situation versus the incremental cost-effectiveness of the prevention program to the baseline (no intervention) situation. Suppose the treatment program costs $100 per routine cocaine user per month while the prevention program costs only $2 per non-user per month. Also suppose that there are societal costs (such as from emergency room visits and incarceration) of $1 per person per month for each rare cocaine user and $50 per person per month for each routine cocaine user. Finally, suppose that the quality-adjusted life-month costs (the utility loss) from being a rare user of cocaine is small, at 0.01 quality adjusted life-months lost for every month of life spent as a rare user of cocaine; but suppose that the quality adjusted life-month loss from being a routine user of cocaine is large, at 0.15 quality adjusted life-months lost for every month of life spent as a routine user of cocaine. Table 5.1 summarizes our input data for our model.

Table 5.1 reflects the typical way we would present the key input assumptions and parameters for a Markov model used to conduct a cost-effectiveness analysis. We would typically accompany such a table with a list of our model equations and initial conditions.

To calculate the overall costs and quality-adjusted utility associated with cocaine use, we can add a fourth and fifth column to our model spreadsheets correspond-ing to the costs and quality-adjusted life-months accumulated over the 120 months of our simulation. Starting with spreadsheet 1 (our baseline, no intervention) scenario, we can add costs into column K and quality-adjusted life months into column L. The value of costs in column K will be equal to the number of peo-ple in each health state, times the cost of being in each health state. Hence, we would multiply 4 million people times the probability of being a rare cocaine user, times the $10 cost of being a rare cocaine user each month, plus 4 million peo-ple times the probability of being a routine cocaine user, times the $500 cost of

Table 5.1 Key input assumptions and parameters for a Markov model used to conduct a cost-effectiveness analysis of prevention or treatment for cocaine use

Parameter	Value
Treatment program cost, per routine cocaine user per month	$100
Prevention program cost, per nonuser of cocaine per month	$2
Costs generated by each rare cocaine user per month	$1
Costs generated by each routine cocaine user per month	$50
Quality-adjusted life-month costs of being a rare user of cocaine per month	0.01
Quality-adjusted life-month costs of being a routine user of cocaine per month	0.15

being a routine cocaine user each month. Hence, the equation in cell K2 should be "=4000000*1*I2+4000000*50*J2." The cell can be left-clicked and dragged down through month 120 to populate the remaining cost estimates for each subsequent month after month 1.

The value of quality-adjusted life-months in column L will be equal to the number of people in each health state, times the quality-adjusted utility of being in each health state. For example, for month 1, we would multiple 4 million people times the probability of each person being a nonuser, times the utility of being a nonuser for 1 month (1 quality-adjusted life-month), plus 4 million people times the probability of each person being a rare user, times the utility of being a rare user for 1 month (1 − 0.01 = 0.99 quality-adjusted life-months), plus 4 million people times the probability of each person being a routine-user, times the utility of being a routine-user for 1 month (1 − 0.15 = 0.85 quality-adjusted life-months). Hence, cell L2 has the equation "=4000000*1*H2+4000000*(1-0.01)*I2+4000000*(1-0.15)*J2." We can left-click and drag this formula down for all 120 months, and we will get a sense of how many quality-adjusted life-months are accumulated in the Los Angeles population over 10 years without any further intervention to curtail the cocaine epidemic. To get a total of the costs and quality-adjusted life-months over the simulated time horizon, we can also insert formulas to calculate the total sum of all costs and quality-adjusted life-months over the simulation period, which we have inserted into the example worksheet in cells M2 and N2, using the formulas "=SUM(K:K)" to calculate the total costs over a 10-year period (column K) and "=SUM(L:L)" to calculate the total quality-adjusted life-months over a 10-year period (column L). To calculate quality-adjusted life-years (QALYs) over the simulation period, we can divide the quality-adjusted life-months by 12. We have placed this calculation into cell O2 of the spreadsheet.

We can copy and paste columns K through N from our baseline model into our treatment spreadsheet and our prevention spreadsheet. We need to add the costs of each intervention to our model, which will be equal to the number of people who are routine cocaine users in a given month times $1,000 in per-month costs for the treatment intervention, and the number of people who are nonusers in a given month times $25 in per-month costs for the prevention intervention. We need to modify our cost columns in column K to include these new costs, such that the cost equation in the treatment spreadsheet row K2 should now be "=4000000*1*I2+4000000 *50*J2+4000000*100*J2," and, similarly, the cost equation in the prevention spreadsheet row K2 should now be "=4000000*1*I2+4000000*50*J2+4000000*2*H2." The spreadsheet uploaded to the book's website provides the complete spreadsheet including these formulas (https://github.com/sanjaybasu/modelinghealthsystems/), which appears in Figure 5.7.

Finally, we can use the costs and QALYs we have estimated to calculate the overall incremental cost-effectiveness ratio (ICER) of the treatment intervention and the prevention intervention. Recalling Chapter 2, the ICER is calculated as:

$$ICER = \frac{\left(New\ Cost - Old\ Cost\right)}{\left(New\ QALYs - Old\ QALYs\right)}.$$ [Equation 5.20]

In our example, we will calculate two ICERs: one for the intervention program and one for the prevention program. The first ICER for the intervention program will be calculated as the cost of the program over the course of 10 years minus the old cost without the program (baseline simulation), all divided by the difference in QALYs with the program minus QALYs without the program. On our spreadsheet, we can create a new sheet to calculate these quantities by typing in an equation that refers to the ICER by referencing each of the other spreadsheets. In our case, if we type "=(Treatment!M2-Baseline!M2)/(Treatment!O2-Baseline!O2)," we refer to the "Treatment" worksheet, as we have called the sheet with our treatment intervention, with the "Treatment!" command (and, specifically, cell M2, containing the cost with treatment, and O2, which contains the QALYs) and the "Baseline" worksheet, as we have called the sheet with our baseline (no intervention) situation, with the

K	L	M	N	O
Cost	Quality-adjusted life months	Total costs	Total quality-adjusted life-months	Total quality-adjusted life years
0	4000000	$ 246,113,348.63	479,166,180.51	39,930,515.04
20000	3999800			
60420	3999563.8			
116181.62	3999302.032			
183218.0548	3999023.145			
258282.5837	3998733.821			
338792.8314	3998439.317			
422704.1323	3998143.735			
508406.5833	3997850.247			

FIGURE 5.7 Cost-effectiveness analysis of a prevention and a treatment intervention for cocaine use, in Excel. The book website contains the Excel spreadsheet corresponding to this example.

"Baseline!" command (and, specifically, the cost cell M2 and QALY cell O2 without treatment). Similarly, we type "=(Prevention!M2-Baseline!M2)/(Prevention!O2-Baseline!O2)," to use the "Prevention" worksheet cost and QALY estimates to compute the ICER of the prevention intervention relative to the baseline of no intervention. We see that, overall, our costs increase from approximately $246 million in the base case to approximately $552 million in the treatment intervention case to approximately $1 billion in the prevention intervention case. Note that because we are integrating costs from the societal perspective, we are including costs to society of not preventing or treatment cocaine use (e.g., incarceration costs) to fairly assess the overall societal costs of cocaine use. We also see that both interventions increase our overall QALYs from 39 million in the baseline no intervention case to about 40 million in the treatment intervention or prevention cases, but with about 34,000 more QALYs saved by the prevention intervention. The overall ICER calculations indicate that both interventions are similarly cost-effective, at between $22,000 and $24,000 per QALY. We can add further complexities to these calculations, such as calculating over longer time-horizons or adding discounting rates, as described in Chapter 2.

CONVENIENT PROPERTIES OF MARKOV MODELS

Markov models have several mathematically convenient properties that are worth illustrating for cases in which a simple hand-calculation is as useful as a spreadsheet-based simulation.

To illustrate these convenient properties, it is worth detailing them by way of example. A classical example is testing for human immunodeficiency virus (HIV). A few years ago, HIV testing was inadequate. There was a large pool of people who had recent HIV infections and could not be detected for several weeks, even though they had the virus in their bloodstream and were infectious to others (i.e., the laboratory tests available could not detect early infection).

We can develop a Markov model to describe the process of HIV testing at one major clinic in San Francisco, where several people visiting the clinic were infected but undetectable. The clinic wanted to minimize the consequences of missing undetectable cases of HIV.

Figure 5.8 provides an illustration of the problem. From the perspective of an uninfected individual patient, there is a probability p each month of becoming infected with HIV and a probability q each month of quitting the clinic (moving away or refusing medical care, a permanent or *terminal* state for the purposes of this problem). Hence, there is a probability $1 - p - q$ that the person will not have become infected and continue coming to the medical clinic. If the patient becomes

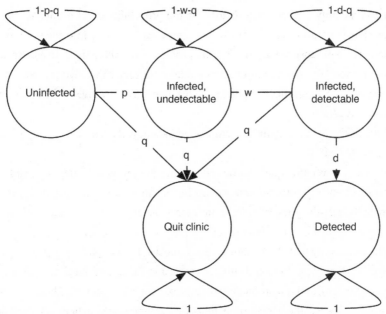

FIGURE 5.8 A Markov model to describe the process of HIV testing at a clinic in San Francisco, where several people visiting the clinic were infected but undetectable. The clinic wanted to minimize the consequences of missing undetectable cases of HIV. There is a probability p each month of becoming infected with HIV, and a probability q each month of quitting the clinic (moving away, or refusing medical care, a permanent or *terminal* state for the purposes of this problem). Hence, there is a probability $1 - p - q$ that the person will not have become infected and continue coming to the medical clinic. If the patient becomes infected, the infection will not be detectable for a certain period of time (the so-called window period). The window period expires with a probability of w each month, and the person continues to have the same probability per month of dropping out of the clinic, so with probability $1 - w - q$ the patient continues in the next month to be infected but not detectable. Once the patient leaves the window period (probability w per month) while still coming to the clinic, they can be detected with a probability d per month. Hence, to the next month without having quit (or having been detected) with probability $1 - d - q$.

infected, the infection will not be detectable for a certain period of time (the so-called window period). The window period expires with a probability of w each month, and the person continues to have the same probability per month of dropping out of the clinic, so with probability $1 - w - q$ the patient continues in the next month to be infected but not detectable. Once the patient leaves the window period (probability w per month) while still coming to the clinic, they can be detected with a probability d per month. Hence, to the next month without having quit (or having been detected) with probability $1 - d - q$.

What is the probability that an uninfected patient will become infected with HIV before quitting the clinic?

We can answer this question just in terms of p and q because of a convenient property of Markov models: the probability that an event happens before any others is the probability of that event divided by the probability of all events *leaving* the given state (i.e., ignoring self-loops). We ignore rates coming into the state for the denominator because we are solving the problem from the perspective of an individual person (i.e., mapping out all possible states they can move to). Hence, the probability that an uninfected patient will become infected with HIV before quitting the clinic is $p/(p + q)$.

What is the probability that an uninfected patient will eventually end up infected and be detected?

We can answer this question by multiplying the probability that an uninfected patient will end up infected and remain in the clinic rather than quitting, by the probability that the patient will end up detectable and remain in the clinic rather than quitting, by the probability that the patient will be detected before quitting.

The probability that the patient ends up infected before quitting is $p/(p + q)$, the probability that the patient ends up detectable and remain in the clinic before quitting is $w/(w + q)$, and the probability that the patient will be detected before quitting is $d/(d + q)$. Hence, the overall probability that an uninfected patient will eventually end up infected and be detected is captured by Equation 5.21:

$$\frac{p}{p+q} \times \frac{w}{w+q} \times \frac{d}{d+q}. \qquad \text{[Equation 5.21]}$$

This solution illustrates how we can "walk along" the length of a Markov model to determine the probability that a person will end up in a particular state. We can also combine information from our Markov model with our learning from Chapter 4, in which we derived queuing models. In Chapter 4, we clarified that the duration of time spent in a given state (a waiting line) was the inverse of the rate of removal from that line. Analogously, a person in a Markov chain would be expected to stay in a given state for a duration of time that amounts to the inverse of the sum of all rates of removal from the state. For example, a person would be expected to stay infected but undetectable for $1/(w + q)$ months because w and q are the rates of removal from the infected but undetectable state.

Knowing this convenient property of Markov models also permits us to answer key questions from the perspective of a public health or healthcare system. For example, suppose the medical clinic decides to start testing people in their clinic at a rate of λ tests per month. What is the expected number of undetectable, infected tests (false-negative tests) that will be recorded by a typical patient who joins the clinic as an uninfected person?

We can reason that a patient who joins the clinic as an uninfected person would first need to become infected before quitting and then would spend a certain amount

of time as an infected but undetectable patient before becoming detectable or quitting. During that time as an infected but undetectable patient, they would be sub-
jected to of λ tests per month according to the problem. Hence, to determine the
number of false-negative tests, we can multiply the probability of becoming infected
before quitting, by the duration of time spent in the infected but undetectable patient
before becoming detectable or quitting, by the rate of testing per month. This is the
expression in Equation 5.22:

$$\frac{p}{p+q} \times \frac{1}{w+q} \times \lambda. \hspace{3cm} \text{[Equation 5.22]}$$

Our example of HIV testing illustrates that describing a problem using a Markov
model can allow us to quickly calculate a number of challenging system-level questions from data that are straightforward to obtain from clinical or medical datasets.
In this example, we could use our model to determine how many false-positive tests
we'd expect based on the rate of testing we choose. We could also use the formulas we
derived to determine how much improved retention in our clinic (reducing the rate
of quitting q) would alter the probability that we eventually detect a patient with HIV
and the number of false-positive tests per patient. Hence, Markov modeling provides
us with a powerful tool to investigate questions about our system and our operations
that would otherwise be difficult to address.

6

PRACTICING TECHNIQUES IN CONTEXT
EXAMPLES FROM FAMINE MANAGEMENT

In this chapter, we will take a brief pause from learning new techniques to reinforce several methods of modeling public health and healthcare systems that we've learned so far. There are at least four major types of modeling that we've detailed in the preceding chapters. First, we dealt with the problem of *resource allocation*, which asks the question: how do we decide which resources to devote to different priority areas? We extended this problem to deal with the allocation of multiple resources in the context of multiple constraints, such as having a limited budget but needing to fulfill many regulatory requirements. Second, we solved *value of information problems*, which ask: how much should we pay to get more information to help us with any given decision? Third, we solved *queuing* problems, which ask: how do we minimize waiting times for a service when demand is higher than supply? Finally, we extended the simple "one-box" queuing model to a multibox *Markov model*, which answers the question: how do we estimate the incidence and prevalence of disease in a population given complex probabilities of getting the disease or being treated for it, and how do we compare the effectiveness and cost-effectiveness of programs to address that disease? In this chapter, we'll practice all four of these key modeling techniques in a common context: designing and evaluating a program to address a famine.

PRACTICE WITH RESOURCE ALLOCATION PROBLEMS

Suppose we work for an international organization that helps provide famine relief internationally. Suppose we are stationed in a region of India providing famine relief services to four states. We have to decide how to best allocate our resources to reduce the health impact of famine.

Problem 1: A Single-Constraint Resource Allocation Decision

To warm up our thinking caps, suppose we have a simple resource allocation problem with only one constraint. Within our service area are populations at high risk of famine in any given year and populations at normal/low risk. Suppose that, out of 100 villages, 30 of them are high risk and the other 70 are normal risk.

Based on data from previous years, we can calculate the typical percent of the time that, if a famine does occur, it occurs in a high-risk population (probability q). Conversely, if a famine does occur, it occurs in the normal/low-risk population with probability $1 - q$.

Suppose that our organization has a limited capacity to detect famine because there are only a few community healthcare workers who can go house-to-house tracking children's nutritional status, thus providing an "early warning" that a famine is developing. Unfortunately, we only have the capacity to send workers to 10 villages due to personnel, budget, and time constraints.

Our task is to decide what fraction of these personnel, call it fraction f, should be devoted to the high-risk villages. For example, if $f = 0.6$, then 60% of all resources to detect a famine will be directed to high-risk villages, with the remaining 40% of the capacity directed to the normal/low-risk villages.

What is the optimal value of f, as a function of q?

This problem is analogous to the resource allocation problem we derived in Chapter 1, in which we tried to maximize "search capacity" to detect a food contamination event at high- and low-risk factories. That problem set the stage for more complex resource allocation problems, being a simple problem with just one resource and just one constraint (one set of resources to distribute).

In this case, we also have one resource (workers trying to detect famine among villages), and we want to maximize the *capture probability* of detecting famine if it is indeed occurring. How can we maximize probability of detecting the famine?

We can first create an equation to express the *objective function* we wish to maximize: the *capture probability*. We can say that the capture probability, the probability of detecting a famine if it is occurring, is equal to the probability of detecting a famine if it is happening in a high-risk population multiplied by the probability that the famine is happening in a high-risk population, plus the probability of detecting a famine if it is happening in a normal-risk population multiplied by the probability that the famine happens in a normal-risk population.

We can estimate that the probability of detecting a famine if it happens in a high-risk population is $f \times 10/30$, because f is the proportion of our resources we dedicate to the high-risk villages, and, if we dedicated all of our resources to the high-risk villages, we would be able to detect the famine in at most 10 of the 30 high-risk villages. Hence fraction f of the 10 out of 30 will be detected. The probability of famine in a high-risk population is q.

Analogously, we can estimate that the probability of detecting a famine if it happens in a normal-risk population is $(1 - f) \times 10/70$, because $(1 - f)$ is the probability of our resources we dedicate to the normal-risk villages, and, if we dedicated all of our resources to the normal-risk villages, we would be able to detect the famine in at most 10 of the 70 normal-risk villages. Hence fraction $(1 - f)$ of the 10 out of 70 will be detected. The probability of famine in a high-risk population is $(1 - q)$.

Overall, therefore, we can say that our capture probability of detecting famine is expressed as Equation 6.1:

$$
\begin{aligned}
P(detection) &= \frac{f \times 10}{30} \times q + \frac{(1-f) \times 10}{70} \times (1-q) \\
&= \frac{1}{3}fq + \frac{1}{7}(1-f)(1-q) \\
&= \frac{1}{3}fq + \frac{1}{7}(1-q) - \frac{1}{7}f(1-q) \\
&= \frac{1}{3}fq - \frac{1}{7}f(1-q) + \frac{1}{7}(1-q) \\
&= \left(\frac{1}{3}q - \frac{1}{7}(1-q)\right)f + \frac{1}{7}(1-q) \\
&= (number) \times f + number.
\end{aligned}
$$

[Equation 6.1]

We can see from our simplification of the equation that the capture probability is a linear equation in f, including a slope and an intercept expression involving variable q. We can reason, from this expression, that the capture probability would be maximized if we chose $f = 1$ (devoting all of our resources to high-risk villages) if the slope is positive. Conversely, the capture probability would be maximized if we chose $f = 0$ (devoting all of our resources to low-risk villages) if the slope is negative. If the slope is equal to zero, it doesn't matter what we choose for variable f; the probability of detecting famine will be the same intercept value of $(1/7) \times (1 - q)$.

Hence, we should set $f = 1$ if the slope is positive, which is expressed as Equation 6.2:

$$
\begin{aligned}
&\left(\frac{1}{3}q - \frac{1}{7}(1-q)\right) > 0 \\
&\left(\frac{1}{3}q + \frac{1}{7}q - \frac{1}{7}\right) > 0 \\
&\frac{10}{21}q > \frac{1}{7} \\
&q > \frac{3}{10}.
\end{aligned}
$$

[Equation 6.2]

Conversely, if $q < 3/10$, we should set $f = 0$.

In plain language terms, if our historical data suggest that more than 30% of famines in the area have been in high-risk villages, we should send all of our workers to those villages. If our historical data suggest that less than 30% of famines in the area have been in high-risk villages, we should send all of our workers to the normal-risk villages. By contrast, if our historical data suggest that exactly 30% of famines have been in high-risk villages, our hands are tied and our choice of where to send the workers will not make any difference.

Our example is a warm-up exercise to remind us of how to derive an expression to optimize a resource allocation decision. It is also unrealistic, in that most of our problems in reality will involve many constraints and will not necessarily descend into a simple solution in which we will put all of our resources into one place or another. The next problem extends the example into a more typical multiconstraint resource allocation situation.

Problem 2: A Multiconstraint Resource Allocation Decision

In the late 2000s, a major relief organization realized that a key strategy to prevent famine was to ensure a sufficient supply of local agricultural crops were produced in an environmentally sustainable manner to help avert famine and simultaneously ensure adequate nutrition for local populations while preserving the quality of farming land for future generations.

In its research, the organization noted that different food production activities had very different impacts on the environment. Table 6.1 summarizes the environmental impact of different types of food production in standard units of farm land devoted to producing each type of food.

Table 6.1 The environmental impact of food production

Food produced	Environmental impact per each land unit of food production					
	Water use (liters)	Emissions (Carbon dioxide kilograms)	Land use (square meters)	Grain use (kilograms for feed)	Calories provided to human consumers (kilocalories)	Protein provided to human consumers (grams)
Beef	15,500	16	7.9	6	2470	7
Chicken	3,900	4.6	6.4	1.8	1650	8.6
Eggs	3,333	5.5	6.7	0	1430	5
Milk	1,000	10.6	9.8	0	610	2
Wheat	1,300	0.8	1.5	0	3400	0.1
Rice	3,400	0	0	0	1300	0

Adapted Bailey, Robert (2011). Growing a better future. Oxford: Oxfam UK. Available at: https://www.oxfam.org/sites/www.oxfam.org/files/growing-a-better-future-010611-en.pdf

As shown in Table 6.1, each unit of land used for beef production uses 15,500 liters of water, produces 16 kilograms of carbon dioxide (cows, apparently, are very flatulent), and provides 2,470 kilocalories of nutrition to the human consumer.

A key goal of the organization's famine prevention programs was to hire local farmers and pay them to produce crops for local consumption. The organization was asked to help these farmers decide what proportion of their farmland to use to grow each of several crops or animals. The goal was to maximize the number of calories produced to prevent famine, but also meet minimum requirements for protein consumption and minimize the ecological footprint of the agricultural production. Suppose our constraints are listed in Table 6.2.

For simplicity, let's also suppose that we only have to optimize our allocation among three food products—beef, chicken, and wheat—and that we want to use all of our land. How can we optimize the distribution of land units so that we distribute a fraction to beef, a fraction to chicken, and a fraction to wheat, maximizing calories and meeting all constraints?

Unlike our first problem, this one would be unduly arduous to solve by hand. We can solve the problem by following the principles of budget optimization that we learned in Chapter 3. We don't have a budget limit but rather a series of environmental limits. We can solve the problem in Excel by entering three key pieces of information into our Excel spreadsheet: (1) the parameters to be modified (in this case, what fraction of land units we dedicate to beef, what fraction to chicken, and what fraction to wheat); (2) the key parameters that we need to consider to meet our constraints and objective function (how much water is used per unit of beef/chicken/wheat, how much carbon dioxide is emitted per unit, how much space is taken up per unit, how much protein is produced per unit, and how many calories are produced per unit); and (3) our *objective function*, which in this case is the number of calories produced, which we want to maximize.

Figure 6.1 provides an example of an Excel spreadsheet with these components entered; this spreadsheet can be downloaded from the book's website (https://github.com/sanjaybasu/modelinghealthsystems/).

Table 6.2 Key constraints for the famine response model

Parameter	Constraint per Unit of Land
Liters of water that can be used	4,000 liters
Kilograms of carbon dioxide that can be emitted	4 kg
Space in square meters	4 square meters
Minimum protein quantity that must be produced	3 grams

	A	B	C	D
1		Beef	Chicken	Wheat
2	Distribution of land units	0.33333333	0.33333333	0.333333333
3	Water use	155500	3900	1300
4	CO2 emitted	16.0	4.6	0.8
5	Space	7.9	6.4	1.5
6	Protein	7.0	8.6	0.1
7	Calories	2,470	1,650	3,400
8				
9	Description	Constraint		Calculated value
10	Water use constraint	4,000	≥	53,566.67
11	CO2 emitted constraint	4	≥	7.13
12	Space constraint	4	≥	5.27
13	Protein minimum requirement	3	≤	5.23
14	Total land fraction used	1	=	1.00
15	Number of calories		MAXIMIZE	2,506.67

FIGURE 6.1 Example of applying multi-constraint optimization in Excel, for the land management problem. An Excel spreadsheet on the book website has the corresponding file available for download.

The top of the spreadsheet declares what we hope to optimize: the fraction of land units to devoted to beef versus chicken versus wheat. We have arbitrarily entered a value of 1/3 as a set of initial conditions, to indicate agnostic equal distribution of land among these three resources, although different starting values adding up to 1 could also be chosen.

The next several rows provide the input parameter data from Table 6.1, indicating how each fraction of land units we dedicate to beef, chicken, or wheat would be expected to impact water use, carbon dioxide emissions, space, and protein production per unit of land.

The final set of rows in Table 6.2 show the constraints. We create a separate column for the calculated values for water, carbon dioxide, space, protein production, and calorie production based on our inputs in column D, cells D10 through D15. Inserting the equations into cells D9 through D15 is the key challenge.

Cell D10 provides the equation for water use and equals the sum of the fraction of land use devoted to beef production times the water use per land unit of beef production, plus the fraction of land use devoted to chicken production times the water use per land unit of chicken production, plus the fraction of land use devoted to wheat production times the water use per land unit of wheat production. This corresponds to equation "=B2*B3+C2*C3+D2*D3" in our spreadsheet in cell D10.

Similarly, cell D11 provides the equation for carbon dioxide emissions and equals the sum of the fraction of land use devoted to beef production times the carbon dioxide emissions per land unit of beef production, plus the fraction of land use devoted to chicken production times the carbon dioxide emissions per land unit of chicken production, plus the fraction of land use devoted to wheat production times the carbon dioxide emissions per land unit of wheat production. This corresponds to equation "=B2*B4+C2*C4+D2*D4" in our spreadsheet in cell D11.

Next, cells D12, D13, and D14 mimic the above cells and provide estimates for the space, protein production, and calorie production.

Cell D15 contains the assumption that we wish to use all of our land. Hence, the sum of the fraction directed to beef, the fraction directed to chicken, and the fraction directed to wheat should equal 1. On Figure 6.1, this corresponds to equation "=B2*B7+C2*C7+D2*D7" in our spreadsheet.

The equations should look like Figure 6.2:

	Description	Constraint		Calculated value
9	Description	Constraint		Calculated value
10	Water use constraint	4000	≥	=B2*B3+C2*C3+D2*D3
11	CO2 emitted constraint	4	≥	=B2*B4+C2*C4+D2*D4
12	Space constraint	4	≥	=B2*B5+C2*C5+D2*D5
13	Protein minimum requirement	3	≤	=B2*B6+C2*C6+D2*D6
14	Total land fraction used	1	=	=B2+C2+D2
15	Number of calories		MAXIMIZE	=B2*B7+C2*C7+D2*D7

FIGURE 6.2 **Equations used for the multi-constraint optimization in Excel, for the land management problem.**

After organizing our model with the parameters, constraints, and objective function, we can next select "Tools" then "Solver" and input our key information. In this case, we want Solver to set the objective of maximizing cell D15, which is the number of calories produced per land unit. We want to do so by changing variable cells B2 through D2 ("B2:D2"), and we need to subject our optimization to the constraints that cell D10 must be less than or equal to B10, D11 less than or equal to B11, D12 less than or equal to B12, D13 greater than or equal to B13, and D14 equal to B14. The Solver window should look like Figure 6.3:

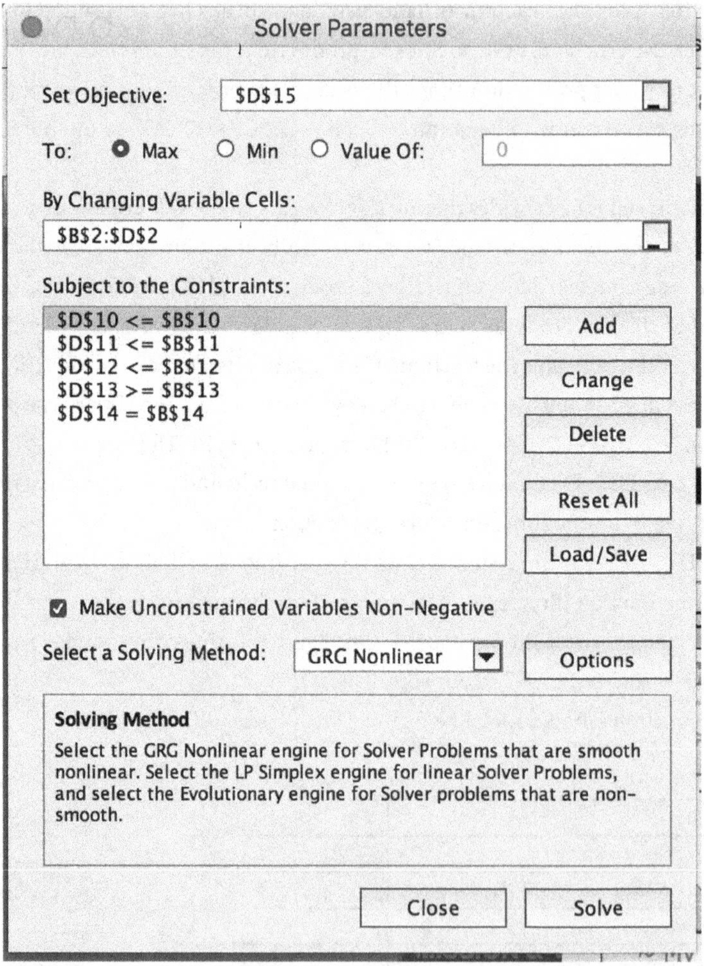

FIGURE 6.3 Solver inputs for the multi-constraint optimization in Excel, for the land management problem.

If we solve for the optimal distribution of resources by clicking "Solve" and "Keep solution," we find that the optimal allocation of land is to devote about 1.2% of land to beef production, 33.2% to chicken, and 65.7% to wheat. We can check that all of our constraints are fulfilled, and we will produce about 2,809 calories per each unit of land in the optimal allocation that meets these constraints.

Problem 3: A Value of Information Problem

A persistent problem in famine management is the challenge of diagnosing children with severe acute malnutrition. Children with the condition can be successfully treated for the disease, but they need to be recognized and sent to dedicated medical care facilities because simple nutritional supplements are typically insufficient to enable their recovery.

A standard test for severe acute malnutrition is a simple paper tape measure that is color-coded and can be wrapped around a child's biceps (a "band test"). The smaller the biceps, the more likely a child is to have severe acute malnutrition. The test is typically performed by mobile community health workers who travel house to house in villages to test children and refer those with very small biceps to local health clinics for further diagnosis and treatment.

Suppose that, for each group of 100 children, about 20 of them in your high-risk villages are truly malnourished and require $50 of treatment each. The band will pick up all 20 of them (suppose it has perfect sensitivity in this population), but the problem is that it will also pick up an additional 10 ("false positives" because of imperfect specificity), wasting an additional $50 of treatment resources per each additional child falsely diagnosed as having severe acute malnutrition.

A $5 prealbumin test has been proposed to be done after the band test to tell us whether the child was a false positive. The test is 90% correct at telling us whether the child was a false positive (10% chance of incorrectly telling us the child was a true positive on their band test) and does not affect true-positive rates (it approves all true-positive children).

Should we pay for the prealbumin test if our objective is to minimize our total cost?

This is a "value of information" problem similar to those we performed in Chapter 2. In this case, we have to determine whether performing the prealbumin test will save costs overall, despite its imperfection. To solve the problem, we can calculate two quantities: the expected cost per child without the prealbumin test, and the expected cost per child with the prealbumin test.

We can draw a decision tree to help us estimate the expected cost per child without the prealbumin test. Figure 6.4 provides the decision tree for this example. In the tree, we have two possible situations: a child either has severe acute malnutrition (20% of the time) or not (80% of the time). If the child has the condition, there is a 100% chance that the band test detects them and a 0% chance that the band test misses them. We then expect to pay $50 in treatment costs for each positive child. If the child does not have the condition, there is a 10 in 80 (12.5% of the time) chance that the test falsely declares them to be positive and a 70 in 80 (87.5% of the time)

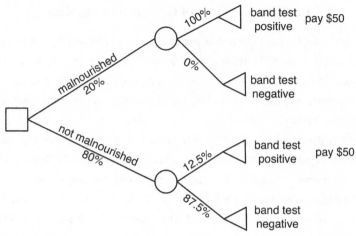

FIGURE 6.4 Decision tree for detecting severe acute malnutrition, without the prealbumin test.

chance that the test correctly declares them to be negative. Among the false-positive children, we expect to pay an additional $50 each.

We can roll back the decision tree such that we calculate the expected cost at the root, which will be the expected cost of the top branch ($0.2 \times 1 \times \$50 + 0.2 \times 0 \times \$0$) plus the expected cost of the bottom branch ($0.8 \times 0.125 \times \$50 + 0.8 \times 0.875 \times \$0$), which equals $15 of expected cost per child.

Next, we can draw an expanded version of this decision tree to help us estimate the expected cost per child with the prealbumin test. The prealbumin test is only performed on those children testing positive, as shown in Figure 6.5, and we pay

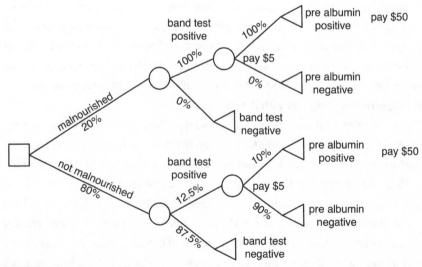

FIGURE 6.5 Decision tree for detecting severe acute malnutrition, with the prealbumin test.

$5 for each prealbumin test. As shown in the figure, among the true positives, the prealbumin test approves all children, and we pay $50 in treatment for these children. Among the false positives, the prealbumin test approves 10% of children for treatment, and we pay $50 for these false positives but not for the other 90% testing negative on the prealbumin test.

We can roll back our decision tree such that we calculate the expected cost at the root, which will be (from top branch to bottom branch): $0.2 \times 1 \times 1 \times (\$50 + \$5) + 0.2 \times 0 \times 0 \times (\$0) + 0.8 \times 0.125 \times 0.1 \times (\$50 + \$5) + 0.8 \times 0.125 \times 0.9 \times (\$5) + 0.8 \times 0.875 \times \$0$, which equals $12 of expected cost per child.

Hence, if cost is our primary consideration, we would do better with the prealbumin test than without it, saving our budget $3 per child on average by purchasing the prealbumin testing service.

Problem 3: A Queuing Problem

Suppose that we are tasked with distributing grain to people we serve, and that the grain storage facility faces long lines. On a typical day, suppose that about 20 people per hour show up to our grain storage facility to pick up food. Suppose that people are very patient and willing to wait in line for approximately 4 hours before leaving (dropping out). Our staff are able to serve about 10 people per hour on average.

Our facility director asks us: how much can we cut down the waiting line and waiting time among people who get service if she provides us the money to hire an additional staff member and serve 12 people per hour instead of just 10?

This question is an example of a typical queuing problem of the sort we solved in Chapter 4. In Chapter 4, we derived two equations to help us solve these types of problems at a steady state: one for queue length and the other for waiting time. Suppose that L is the steady-state value for the length of the waiting line and that δ (delta) is the demand to enter the line per unit time, σ (sigma) is the supply of services per unit time, μ (mu) is the drop-out rate from the line, and W is the duration of waiting in line among people who get service. Then, from Chapter 4, we had the following two equations:

$$L = \frac{(\delta - \sigma)}{\mu}. \qquad\qquad \text{[Equation 6.3]}$$

$$\frac{\sigma}{\delta} = e^{-\mu W}. \qquad\qquad \text{[Equation 6.4]}$$

We can use these two equations to answer the facility director's question. First, we can solve for the typical waiting line length and typical duration of waiting in line until people get service, given our current rate of providing service to 10 people per hour. We can say that our demand δ is 20 people per hour, our service rate σ is 10 people per hour, and the drop-out rate is the inverse of the duration of time people are willing to wait in line; hence, $\mu = 1/4$ hours or 0.25 hours^{-1}.

Using Equation 6.3, we can then solve that $L = (20 - 10)/(0.25) = 40$ people in the waiting line (or queue) at any given time. Similarly, using Equation 6.4, we can solve that $W = (1/0.25) \, ln(20/10) = 2.8$ as the hours a typical person who gets service waits in line, on average.

What if we add the new staff member? Then our rate of service, σ, shifts to 12 people per hour and so $L = (20 - 12)/(0.25) = 32$ people in the waiting line at any given time. Hence, we cut the length of the line by 8 people. Similarly, $W = (1/0.25) \, ln(20/12) = 2.0$ hours a typical person who gets service would wait in line after we get the additional staff member. Hence, we cut 0.8 hours, which is about 48 minutes from the waiting time among those getting service.

Here's a critical question: how many people would have dropped out from having the old number of staff, but would no longer drop out with the new, higher number of staff? The answer would be 0.25/hour (rate of dropping out) $\times$ 0.8 hours = 0.2 persons (or a fifth of a person, statistically speaking).

Problem 4: Markov Modeling

Suppose we have a presentation at the United Nations next Monday and need to convince the "big wigs" that our program is making an impact on malnutrition.

We have a limited amount of data available to us to assess the impact of the program on individual children. Suppose that children can be in one of three possible states: healthy, mildly malnourished, or severely malnourished. Normally, without our program, about 5% of children per month go from being healthy to being mildly malnourished (none go straight to severe malnutrition); another 20% of children per month with mild malnutrition become healthy again through natural recovery processes, while 10% of those with mild malnutrition become severely malnourished per month; finally, 30% of children per month go from severe to mildly malnourished through natural recovery, and the rest stay in severe malnutrition (none go straight back to healthy).

Our program treats children with severe malnutrition. It increases the probability of transitioning from severely malnourished to healthy, from 0% per month to 50% per month. The other 50% of severely malnourished children in the area go from severely malnourished to mildly malnourished each month.

The United Nations officials will ask you: "What's the impact of the program on the prevalence of severe malnutrition?"

To answer this question, we can create a Markov model following the principles and strategies we detailed in Chapter 5.

As with every Markov model, we start by first drawing the model diagram shown in Figure 6.6. Here, we draw the diagram before our intervention has been introduced.

In Figure 6.6, we first drew the three possible states, then the arrows connecting each possible state to each other possible state. We then filled in the probabilities per month on these arrows using the information provided in the problem. Last, we solved for the value of "self-loop" probabilities by reasoning that a person has probability 1 that they will either convert to another state or stay in the same state from month to month; hence, 1 minus the rates of flow out of a state is the value of the probability of remaining within a given state from one month to the next. Note that we ignore mortality for our modeling example here, but can add in death as a fourth state to be more realistic.

Next, we write down our equations for this Markov model. In the pre-intervention case, we can use the reasoning from Chapter 5 to write down a series of steady-state equations that reflect the probability of being in a state in terms of the probability of coming into that state from one of the three states to the state being examined. A fourth equation is the equation that tells us that the probability of being in any

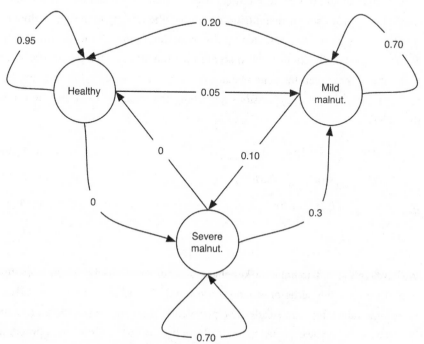

FIGURE 6.6 A Markov model of the malnutrition, without the treatment program.

given state is equal to 1, meaning that no person can escape the model, and the three states comprehensively describe all possible states of being with respect to our problem. These expressions are shown in Equations 6.5 through 6.9.

$$p_{healthy} = 0.95p_{healthy} + 0.2p_{mild} + 0p_{severe}$$ [Equation 6.5]

$$p_{mild} = 0.05p_{healthy} + 0.7p_{mild} + 0.3p_{severe}$$ [Equation 6.6]

$$p_{severe} = 0p_{healthy} + 0.1p_{mild} + 0.7p_{severe}$$ [Equation 6.7]

$$p_{healthy} + p_{mild} + p_{severe} = 1.$$ [Equation 6.8]

We can solve these equations by hand, or (as we will see in a moment) solve them using Excel, giving the solution that $p_{healthy} = 0.75$, $p_{mild} = 0.1875$, and $p_{severe} = 0.0625$. Hence, before our intervention, there is about a 6% chance of being severely malnourished. In a village of 100,000 children, we would expect the long-term steady-state prevalence of severe malnutrition to be $100,000 \times p_{severe} = 6,250$ children.

How much difference will our program make to this prevalence? We can account for the change in the malnutrition epidemic by redrawing our Markov model to account for the higher probability of becoming healthy from severe malnutrition or reverting to mild malnutrition from severe malnutrition, as shown in Figure 6.7.

Note that, in addition to accounting for the increased probability per month of transitioning from severe malnutrition to either the healthy or mildly malnourished state, we have also accounted for the reduction in the "self-loop" probability of staying severely malnourished to account for the fact that the total probability of leaving or staying in the state remains at the value of 1. From the diagram, we can write the new set of expressions describing the steady state as Equations 6.9 through 6.12.

$$p_{healthy} = 0.95p_{healthy} + 0.2p_{mild} + \mathbf{0.5}p_{severe}$$ [Equation 6.9]

$$p_{mild} = 0.05p_{healthy} + 0.7p_{mild} + \mathbf{0.5}p_{severe}$$ [Equation 6.10]

$$p_{severe} = 0p_{healthy} + 0.1p_{mild} + \mathbf{0}p_{severe}$$ [Equation 6.11]

$$p_{healthy} + p_{mild} + p_{severe} = 1.$$ [Equation 6.12]

We have highlighted, in bold, the key changes to our equations due to our intervention. If we solve this series of equations, we will find an estimate of $p_{severe} = 0.0164$. Hence, the new long-term steady-state prevalence of severe malnutrition after our intervention would be expected to be $100,000 \times p_{severe} = 1,640$ children. Our program

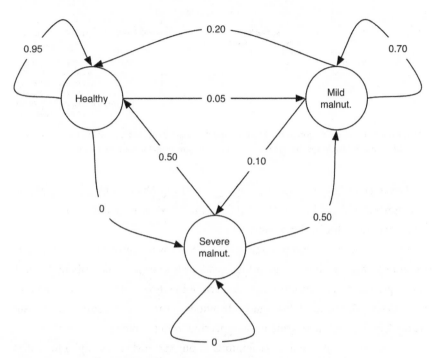

FIGURE 6.7 **A Markov model of the malnutrition, with the treatment program.**

has reduced the long-term prevalence of severe malnutrition by more than 4,000 children.

What if we wanted to solve for periods other than the long-term steady-state? And what if we wanted to assess the cost-effectiveness of our program? Suppose we have the data available to us in Table 6.3 to detail the cost and utility, in quality-adjusted life-months, of being malnourished. What would be the incremental cost-effectiveness ratio of our intervention as compared to the baseline case of not having any intervention?

Table 6.3 Key parameters for estimating the cost-effectiveness of the malnutrition intervention

Parameter	Value
Cost of mild malnutrition to society (e.g., economic burden on family) per month	$10
Cost of severe malnutrition to society per month	$25
Cost of treating severe malnutrition per month	$50
Quality-adjusted life-month utility loss from mild malnutrition	0.1
Quality-adjusted life-month utility loss from severe malnutrition	0.3

	A	B	C	D	E	F	G	H	I	J
				Coming from:			Time (month)	P(healthy)	P(mild)	P(severe)
1	Transition matrix									
2			healthy	mild	severe		1	1	0	0
3		healthy	0.95	0.2	0		2	0.95	0.05	0
4	Entering into:	mild	0.05	0.7	0.3		3	0.9125	0.0825	0.005
5		severe	0	0.1	0.7		4	0.883375	0.104875	0.01175
6							5	0.86018125	0.12110625	0.0187125
7							6	0.84139344	0.13339719	0.02520938
8							7	0.8260032	0.14301052	0.03098628
9							8	0.81330515	0.15070341	0.03599145

FIGURE 6.8 Implementation of the Markov model of malnutrition treatment in Excel. An Excel spreadsheet on the book website has the corresponding file available for download.

We can create an Excel spreadsheet to solve this problem, which is diagrammed in Figure 6.8 and can be downloaded from the book's website (https://github.com/sanjaybasu/modelinghealthsystems/).

As in Chapter 5, we start programming the Markov model by first creating a transition matrix in which we convert the equations into a matrix describing the probability per month of transitioning from each of the three states to each of the other three states. We can check that our probabilities in each column sum to 1 to ensure we don't have people appearing or disappearing from the model.

Second, we create a column (column G in our spreadsheet example) to indicate the *time steps* of the model. Here, we model in monthly time steps over a 10-year *planning horizon*, or 120 months. We populate this column by putting the number "1" in the first row of numbers (cell G2), then the formula "=1+G2" in the next cell, and clicking and dragging the bottom right of the formula cell to populate the rest of the numbers automatically.

Third, we set the *initial conditions* for the model. We have arbitrarily assumed that the probability of being healthy is 1 before the famine, and there are no mild or severe cases of malnutrition; hence, the first row of probabilities is set to 1 for $p_{healthy}$, 0 for p_{mild}, and 0 for p_{severe}. But, as we found in Chapter 5, these initial conditions only affect our pre–steady-state outcomes, and the steady-state solution remains dependent only on the transition matrix. Hence, no matter what initial conditions we choose, the steady-state solution will remain the same.

Fourth, we fill in the key equations corresponding to the probabilities of being in each state in the next month given the probabilities of being in a given state the previous month. Here, we insert Equations 6.5 through 6.8 into Excel, referring to our transition matrix to provide the transition matrix values for the probability of moving between states. For example, the probability of being healthy in month 2 is "=C$3*H2+D$3*I2+E$3*J2," where the dollar signs tell Excel to refer consistently to values in the transition matrix and not shift those values when we later click and drag our equations down to subsequent months.

The spreadsheet equations should look like those in Figure 6.9.

	G	H	I	J
1	**Time (month)**	**P(healthy)**	**P(mild)**	**P(severe)**
2	1	1	0	0
3	=G2+1	=C$3*H2+D$3*I2+E$3*J2	=C$4*H2+D$4*I2+E$4*J2	=C$5*H2+D$5*I2+E$5*J2

FIGURE 6.9 **Time and state equations for the Markov model of malnutrition treatment in Excel.**

Once we click and drag the equations down to all cells for all time points, we can have the model populate the remaining months of values for the probabilities, which should give us the solutions reported above for steady-state probabilities.

Next, we can add in the cost-effectiveness analysis. First, we create a duplicate version of our model by right-clicking the bottom left of the spreadsheet, on the tab that says "Sheet 1" by default, or "Baseline" in our spreadsheet, and creating a copy of the entire spreadsheet (click "move to end" and check the "create a copy" box). On the copy of the spreadsheet, we can modify the transition matrix to correspond to the new post-intervention values of the transition matrix, giving us the new probabilities of being in each state after our intervention (which changes column E3 through E6 to values of 0.5, 0.5, and 0, respectively, as per Equations 6.9 through 6.12).

Now to add a cost-effectiveness analysis, we need to add the costs and quality-adjusted life-months for both our baseline (pre-intervention) and post-intervention situations. In the "baseline" tab, we can add in the costs to society of both mild and severe malnutrition (Table 6.3) in column K. For a population of 100,000 children, we would add to cell K2 the equation "=100000*10*I2+100000*25*J2," which is the population size multiplied by the $10 cost of mild malnutrition to society, multiplied by the probability that each child is mildly malnourished, plus the population size multiplied by the $25 cost of severe malnutrition to society, multiplied by the probability that the child is severely malnourished. Similarly, we can add the quality-adjusted life-months gained in column L by inserting equation "=100000*1*H2+100000* (1−0.1)*I2+100000*(1−0.3)*J2" into cell L2. This adds the population size multiplied by the quality-adjusted life-month utility value of being healthy (value of 1) times the probability of being healthy, plus the population size multiplied by the quality-adjusted life-month utility value of being mildly malnourished (value of 1 minus 0.1 per Table 6.3) times the probability of being mildly malnourished, plus the population size multiplied by the quality-adjusted life-month utility value of being severely malnourished (value of 1 minus 0.3) times the probability of being severely malnourished. We can left-click and drag these two equations down columns K and L, respectively, to populate all 10 years of time in the model. In our example spreadsheet, we have also added the total costs and total quality-adjusted life-months in cells M2 and N2. We did so by inserting the expressions "=SUM(K:K)" into M2

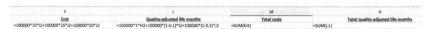

FIGURE 6.10 **Equations used to calculate incremental cost-effectiveness for the Markov model of malnutrition treatment in Excel.**

for adding costs and "=SUM(L:L)" into N2 for adding quality-adjusted life-months. We also calculated the quality-adjusted life-years (QALYs) in cell O2 by dividing the quality-adjusted life-month sum by 12. Note that we have not discounted the sum of costs or sum of quality-adjusted life-months, but we could do so by dividing each month's costs and quality-adjusted life-months by $(1 + \text{discount rate})^{\wedge}(\text{years passed})$ (i.e., $1.03^{\wedge}(6/12)$) if we are discounting the results by 3% per year and we are computing the costs and quality-adjusted life-months corresponding to month 6. Without discounting, our equations for costs and quality-adjusted life-months look like Figure 6.10.

Next, we can copy and paste columns K through O from our "Baseline" tab into our "Intervention" tab to compute the costs and quality-adjusted life-months after our intervention. We need to add in costs of our intervention itself, so, in the cost column K, we modify the equation to include the cost of treating severe malnutrition per month, modifying the formula in K2 to "=100000*10*I2+100000*25*J2+100000* 50*J2." Note that if not every child gets treatment (i.e., imperfect access to therapy), we could modify this equation further to multiply the cost by less than 100,000 and replace the population size multiplied by the probability J2 of being severely malnourished with an alternative estimate of the number of children we are actually able to serve per month.

Finally, we can calculate the incremental cost-effectiveness ratio (ICER) of our intervention as compared to the baseline condition of no intervention. We have created a new spreadsheet by clicking the "+" button to the right of the tabs at the bottom of the screen and naming it "ICER." We have then calculated the difference in costs as "=(Intervention!M2-Baseline!M2)," where we refer to the spreadsheet name followed by an explanation point to tell Excel to refer to the corresponding sheet, in which M2 is the 10-year cost total. We have also calculated the difference in QALYs as "=(Intervention!O2-Baseline!O2)." Finally, the ICER is the quotient of the difference in costs divided by the difference in QALYs, which in this case is a negative number: −$389 per QALY saved. We can see that the negative is being produced because our intervention situation actually produces less costs than our baseline condition. In other words, our intervention averts so many cases of severe acute malnutrition that it actually saves society money. This is one of those rare circumstances in which a public health intervention is cost-saving while also producing a gain in QALYs.

PART THREE

Simulations

7

MODELING IN *R*

In previous chapters, we implemented our models in spreadsheets for several reasons: (1) spreadsheet are straightforward to work with and do not require extensive knowledge of programming; (2) spreadsheets are easy to communicate with among people with varying levels of expertise; (3) spreadsheets are convenient for optimization problems, given the availability of prepackaged Solver algorithms; and (4) spreadsheets are commonly used for modeling in the world of business management, nonprofit organization budgeting, consulting, and academia. But spreadsheets have their limitations, particularly when we want to model large populations, long periods of time, or complex situations in which we have many states or conditions and lots of equations. For larger scale models where we desire more flexibility than can be offered by a spreadsheet, the free statistical program *R* provides a straightforward approach to modeling and has the advantages of being free, fast, available on any operating system, commonly used, and widely supported by an online community that helps users who get stuck. In this chapter, we provide a detailed introduction to using *R* that will be useful for the more advanced modeling methods we introduce and practice in Chapters 8 through 11.

SETTING UP *R*

R is supported by a vast online support system called the Comprehensive R Archive Network (CRAN). The easiest way to get started using *R* is to download the *R* program by simply doing a web search for the letter "R," and opening the website for CRAN, which has a "Download" page where *R* can be downloaded and installed for any system (https://cran.r-project.org/).

For our purposes, *R* can be thought of as analogous to the engine of a car: it's a powerful tool that we will use, but unless we're mechanics, we don't want to interfere with its underlying components. Just as we would sit comfortably in front of a dashboard in a car and use our steering wheel and pedals to control the engine, we also want a comfortable dashboard to take our commands and run it through the engine of *R*. Hence, we want to have an interface that's easier to use than just the standard *R* command line. We prefer *RStudio*, which is free and one of the most popular interfaces that will accept our commands, put them into the engine in *R*, and provide a nice output for us. If we web search "RStudio," a free download is available for any operating system (https://www.rstudio.com/products/rstudio/download/). For the purposes of this book, the "Desktop" not the "Server" version of *RStudio* should be installed.

Once we have installed both *R* and *RStudio*, we can open *RStudio* itself, which looks like Figure 7.1.

RStudio will send our commands to the engine of *R* and retrieve the output for us; hence, we do not need to open *R* itself separately (we just leave it on our hard drive). At the top left of Figure 7.1, we can see a white square with a "+" sign, which we click to start a new "R Script." This opens a blank page for us to use. *RStudio* is organized into four sections by default, with a "Code" window that we just opened to type in commands; a "Console" window that appears in the top right of Figure 7.1 (but may be located on the bottom left corner of some systems), which tell us what the engine is doing and provides output to our

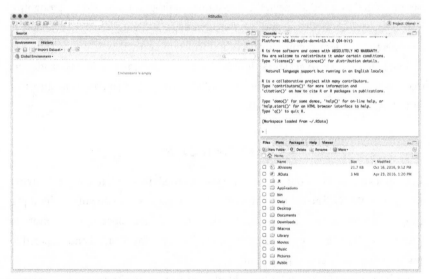

FIGURE 7.1 Screenshot of *RStudio*. At the top left of the figure, we can see a white square with a "+" sign, which we should click to start a new "R Script". This opens a blank page for us to use. *RStudio* is organized into four sections by default, with a "Code" window that we just opened to type in commands; a "Console" window that appears in the top right of the figure (but maybe located on the bottom left corner of some systems), which tell us what the engine is doing and provides our output to our commands; a "Workspace" (bottom left of the figure, but occasionally top right on some systems) that shows us the names of our parameters and datasets, and a window with several tabs that allows us to find files, view plots, get help, and install packages.

commands; a "Workspace" (bottom left of Figure 7.1, but occasionally top right on some systems) that shows us the names of our parameters and datasets, and a window with several tabs that allows us to find files, view plots, get help, and install packages. Packages in *R* are like apps on a smartphone; if we want extra features, we can install from the Internet a package produced by expert users to save us time for common tasks.

To get started in *R*, we should learn a few common resources to help us whenever we have questions. We recommend Quick-R, a popular, free webpage that explains useful commands in *R* such as how to import data, change directories, make plots, save our results, and so on (http://www.statmethods.net/).

USEFUL *R* COMMANDS

For the purposes of solving public health or health system problems, we need to become familiar with a few key commands in *R* that are useful for modeling. The code that we provide here can also be downloaded from this book's website (https://github.com/sanjaybasu/modelinghealthsystems/). Code files in *R* end with the extension ".R."

First, in the code window (the blank page that we created at the upper left), let's see how *R* works as a calculator. We can type in 1 + 2 in the code window, and then click the "Run" button at the top right of the window, as shown in Figure 7.2.

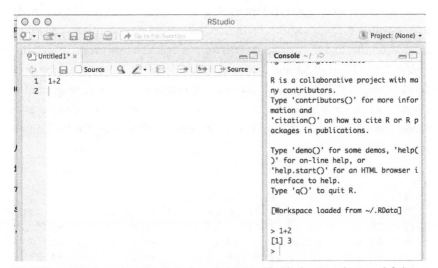

FIGURE 7.2 **Simple commands in R.** In the code window (the blank page at the upper left that we created), we can type in 1+2, and then click the "Run" button at the top right of the window, which looks like a green arrow pointing out of a rectangle.

When we click "Run," we see that *R* provides us with the output in the Console window that looks like this:

```
> 1+2
[1]  3
```

This output shows us three things: (1) our command (which follows the > sign) was to add 1 plus 2; (2) we had one result (shown as [1]); and (3) the result is the number 3. Note that we can put our cursor on the end of a line of code and click "Run" to transfer just that line of code to *R*, or we can highlight a few lines and click "Run" to run several lines of code at once. We can store the value as a variable *test* by typing the command: `test=1+2`. *R* will then store the number "3" as variable *test*. If we type *test* and click "Run," *R* will output a single result, the number 3:

```
> test=1+2
> test
[1]  3
```

For modeling purposes, we often wish to store long lists of numbers, or *vectors*, rather than just a single number. For example, let's use the `repeat` command to create a vector of 10 zeros: rep(0,10)

```
> rep(0,10)
[1]  0  0  0  0  0  0  0  0  0  0
```

As another example, suppose that we want to count every month in a Markov model from month 1 through month 120. In Excel, we would need to make a cell in our spreadsheet that had the number "1" (let's say in cell A1), then create an equation such as "=1+A1" in cell A2, and drag that formula down 120 cells to create the numbers 1 through 120. In *R*, creating vectors is as simple as writing the starting number, a colon, and the ending number. For example, suppose we type 1:120 in the code window, and then click the "Run" button. We would get the output in the Console window that looks like this:

```
> 1:120
  [1]   1   2   3   4   5   6   7   8   9  10  11  12  13  14   15   16   17
 [18]  18  19  20  21  22  23  24  25  26  27  28  29  30  31   32   33   34
 [35]  35  36  37  38  39  40  41  42  43  44  45  46  47  48   49   50   51
 [52]  52  53  54  55  56  57  58  59  60  61  62  63  64  65   66   67   68
 [69]  69  70  71  72  73  74  75  76  77  78  79  80  81  82   83   84   85
 [86]  86  87  88  89  90  91  92  93  94  95  96  97  98  99  100  101  102
```

```
[103] 103 104 105 106 107 108 109 110 111 112 113 114 115 116
117 118 119
[120] 120
```

This output shows us that *R* has quickly produced all the numbers from 1 through 120. The square brackets on the left help us keep track of which position in the vector is occupied by a given number whenever our vector spills over from one line of the console window to the next line; for example, position 18 in the vector is the number 18, and position 35 in the vector is position 35.

R will let us easily save vectors in order to use them later. For example, if we type into our code window the command: months = 1:120, then what we're doing is creating a vector named *months* which contains all the numbers from 1 to 120. If we click "Run" then the output looks like this:

```
> months=1:120
```

In other words, *R* has not done anything but stored the output under the name *months*. The word "months" should now appear in our "Workspace" window. If we later want to do anything with the vector months, we can type in the name *months* rather than having to retype the underlying numbers. For example, suppose we wanted to create another vector called *years*. We could just type into our code window: years = months/12. When we click "Run" we see that years has been stored, and if we just type the word "years" into the code window and click "Run," we will get the output:

```
> years=months/12
> years
 [1]  0.08333333  0.16666667  0.25000000  0.33333333  0.41666667
 [6]  0.50000000  0.58333333  0.66666667  0.75000000  0.83333333
[11]  0.91666667  1.00000000  1.08333333  1.16666667  1.25000000
[16]  1.33333333  1.41666667  1.50000000  1.58333333  1.66666667
[21]  1.75000000  1.83333333  1.91666667  2.00000000  2.08333333
[26]  2.16666667  2.25000000  2.33333333  2.41666667  2.50000000
[31]  2.58333333  2.66666667  2.75000000  2.83333333  2.91666667
[36]  3.00000000  3.08333333  3.16666667  3.25000000  3.33333333
[41]  3.41666667  3.50000000  3.58333333  3.66666667  3.75000000
[46]  3.83333333  3.91666667  4.00000000  4.08333333  4.16666667
[51]  4.25000000  4.33333333  4.41666667  4.50000000  4.58333333
[56]  4.66666667  4.75000000  4.83333333  4.91666667  5.00000000
[61]  5.08333333  5.16666667  5.25000000  5.33333333  5.41666667
[66]  5.50000000  5.58333333  5.66666667  5.75000000  5.83333333
[71]  5.91666667  6.00000000  6.08333333  6.16666667  6.25000000
[76]  6.33333333  6.41666667  6.50000000  6.58333333  6.66666667
```

```
[81]   6.75000000  6.83333333  6.91666667  7.00000000  7.08333333
[86]   7.16666667  7.25000000  7.33333333  7.41666667  7.50000000
[91]   7.58333333  7.66666667  7.75000000  7.83333333  7.91666667
[96]   8.00000000  8.08333333  8.16666667  8.25000000  8.33333333
[101]  8.41666667  8.50000000  8.58333333  8.66666667  8.75000000
[106]  8.83333333  8.91666667  9.00000000  9.08333333  9.16666667
[111]  9.25000000  9.33333333  9.41666667  9.50000000  9.58333333
[116]  9.66666667  9.75000000  9.83333333  9.91666667 10.00000000
```

We see here that R has created a vector named *years* and has divided all elements of the vector *months* by 12 to get the values of time in units of years. You can imagine this is equivalent to listing all the months in one column of Excel and then creating a second column that divided the first column by 12.

We can also create vectors by using the concatenate command, which means we can type numbers into a vector manually; for example, suppose we want a vector called *testvector* that contains the numbers 1, 3, 6, and 8. We can just type testvector = c(1,3,6,8), where "c" with parentheses tells us to concatenate (link together) the four numbers in a vector.

```
> testvector=c(1,3,6,8)
> testvector
[1] 1 3 6 8
```

We can pull up any element of a vector by calling the vector name and the element number in square brackets. For example, if we want the third element of *testvector*, we can type: testvector[3] and get:

```
> testvector[3]
[1] 6
```

R makes it convenient to identify the individual values within a vector. For example, suppose we want to identify what the value of the vector *years* is in month 70. We can simply type the command: years[months==70], which means "tell us which value of the vector years corresponds to the point at which the vector months is equal to a value of 70." Note that the command includes a double equal sign "==" not a single equal sign; a single equal sign would tell R to set the value of a variable or vector to a particular value, whereas a double equal sign means "go look for when this variable or vector equals this value." We get the output:

```
> years[months==70]
[1] 5.833333
```

Similarly, suppose we want to know all values of the vector *years* for which the variable months is greater than 100. We would type the command: years[months>100] and get:

```
> years[months>100]
 [1] 8.416667  8.500000  8.583333  8.666667  8.750000  8.833333
8.916667
 [8] 9.000000  9.083333  9.166667  9.250000  9.333333  9.416667
9.500000
[15] 9.583333  9.666667  9.750000  9.833333  9.916667 10.000000
```

Suppose we just want to pull out all values of the vector *years* that are between 5 and 10. We can type the command: years[(years>5)&(years<10)]. This tells *R* to look into the vector *years* and look for values greater than 5 that are also (&) less than a value of 10. Alternatively, if we want "or," then we can include the vertical line "|" in place of the ampersand "&" to find all years greater than 5 or less than 10. If we use the "and" command, we get:

```
> years[(years>5)&(years<10)]
 [1] 5.083333  5.166667  5.250000  5.333333  5.416667  5.500000
5.583333
 [8] 5.666667  5.750000  5.833333  5.916667  6.000000  6.083333
6.166667
[15] 6.250000  6.333333  6.416667  6.500000  6.583333  6.666667
6.750000
[22] 6.833333  6.916667  7.000000  7.083333  7.166667  7.250000
7.333333
[29] 7.416667  7.500000  7.583333  7.666667  7.750000  7.833333
7.916667
[36] 8.000000  8.083333  8.166667  8.250000  8.333333  8.416667
8.500000
[43] 8.583333  8.666667  8.750000  8.833333  8.916667  9.000000
9.083333
[50] 9.166667  9.250000  9.333333  9.416667  9.500000  9.583333
9.666667
[57] 9.750000  9.833333  9.916667
```

Just as we can create vectors in *R*, we can also create matrices, such as transition matrices for Markov models. To create a matrix, we create a vector and then tell *R* to organize the vector into a series of columns and rows. For example, suppose we want a matrix to look like this:

$$
\begin{bmatrix} 0.995 & 0.15 & 0.02 \\ 0.005 & 0.826 & 0.04 \\ 0 & 0.024 & 0.94 \end{bmatrix}.
$$ [Equation 7.1]

We could type in the full vector of numbers, left to right and top to bottom, and use the matrix command in *R* to turn that vector into a matrix named *testmatrix*: `testmatrix = matrix(c(0.995,0.15,0.02,0.005,0.826,0.04,0, 0.024,0.94),ncol=3,byrow=TRUE)`. In this command, matrix tells *R* to turn the vector into a matrix, "c" tells *R* what numbers to put into the vector, "ncol" tells *R* how many columns the matrix should be, and "byrow=TRUE" tells *R* that we want the vector to be read into the matrix row by row (so that 0.995 is followed by 0.15 in row 1, not by 0.005):

```
> testmatrix = matrix(c(0.995,0.15,0.02,0.005,0.826,0.04,0,0.
024,0.94),ncol=3,byrow=TRUE)
> testmatrix
      [,1]   [,2]  [,3]
[1,]  0.995  0.150 0.02
[2,]  0.005  0.826 0.04
[3,]  0.000  0.024 0.94
```

A MARKOV MODEL IN *R*

Let's recreate our Markov model of the Los Angeles cocaine epidemic from Chapter 5 in *R* instead of in Excel. To recall, our goal was to model how nonusers of cocaine may become rare users and routine users, as shown in Figure 7.3.

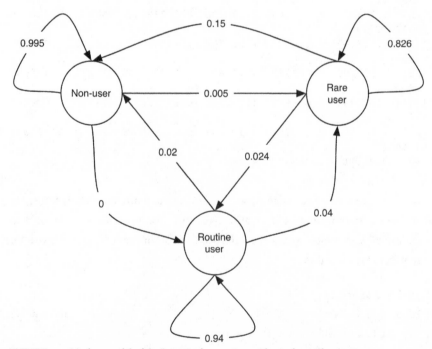

FIGURE 7.3 **Markov model of the Los Angeles cocaine epidemic from Chapter 5.**

To create this Markov model, we need the same three components of the model as we did in Excel: a transition matrix, a set of initial conditions, and a series of vectors (which were columns in Excel). The transition matrix is the same at the one shown earlier: it is the matrix showing us the probability of moving among the three states in our model; hence, we can simply adopt the command from earlier:

```
transition = matrix(c(0.995,0.15,0.02,0.005,0.826,0.04,0,0.02
4,0.94),ncol=3,byrow=TRUE)
```

The initial conditions can be set such that we have a probability of 1 of being a nonuser at the start and probabilities of 0 of being a rare user or a routine user at the start. We can create three vectors that will be empty at the start of the model and that we will fill in for every month of our simulation. We do that by typing the commands:

```
timesteps =120
pnon = rep(0,timesteps)
prare = rep(0,timesteps)
proutine = rep(0,timesteps)
```

Among these commands, `timesteps` tells us how many periods of time (in this case, months) will be simulated in the model. The subsequent commands create vectors of 120 zeros to fill in later. We want to fill in the first value of the pnon vector with the value "1" to correspond to the initial conditions. We do that by typing:

```
pnon[1] = 1
```

Note that by using a single equals sign, not a double equals sign, we have assigned a value of 1 to the *pnon* vector at time step 1. We can check by typing "pnon," which now outputs:

```
> pnon
 [1] 1 0 0 0 0 0 0 0 0 0 0 0 0 0 0 0 0 0 0 0 0 0 0 0 0 0 0 0 0 0 0 0
 0 0 0 0
[33] 0 0 0 0 0 0 0 0 0 0 0 0 0 0 0 0 0 0 0 0 0 0 0 0 0 0 0 0 0 0 0 0
 0 0 0 0
[65] 0 0 0 0 0 0 0 0 0 0 0 0 0 0 0 0 0 0 0 0 0 0 0 0 0 0 0 0 0 0 0 0
 0 0 0 0
[97] 0 0 0 0 0 0 0 0 0 0 0 0 0 0 0 0 0 0 0 0 0 0 0 0
```

We can see here that the first vector value has been changed to "1" and the remaining components remain as values of zero.

Now we need to update the model to calculate the probabilities of being a nonuser, rare user, or routine user for subsequent months. To do so, let's recall that the Markov model's equations can be expressed in the following form with matrix multiplication:

$$\begin{bmatrix} 0.995 & 0.15 & 0.02 \\ 0.005 & 0.826 & 0.04 \\ 0 & 0.024 & 0.94 \end{bmatrix} \begin{bmatrix} p_{non}(t-1) \\ p_{rare}(t-1) \\ p_{routine}(t-1) \end{bmatrix} = \begin{bmatrix} p_{non}(t) \\ p_{rare}(t) \\ p_{routine}(t) \end{bmatrix}. \qquad \text{[Equation 7.2]}$$

We can first create a vector for what the values of p_{non}, p_{rare}, and $p_{routine}$ were at a given time $t - 1$ and then multiply that vector by the transition matrix to get the values at time t. For example, let's create a vector called *priorstate* which will consistent of the values of p_{non}, p_{rare}, and $p_{routine}$ at month 1. We can write the code priorstate = c(pnon[1],prare[1], proutine[1]), which would mean that the *priorstate* vector is the first value of vectors *pnon, prare,* and *proutine*:

```
> priorstate =c(pnon[1],prare[1],proutine[1])
> priorstate
[1] 1 0 0
```

What will be the values of p_{non}, p_{rare}, and $p_{routine}$ at the next time point? Based on Equation 7.2, it would be the value of our transition matrix multiplied by the value of our current state vector. In R, while regular multiplication is conducted by typing the asterisk (*) symbol, matrix multiplication is conducted just by wrapping the asterisk in parentheses (%*%). We can see that multiplying the transition matrix by the current state matrix (the probability of being in each state in month 1) provides us with the probability of being in each state during month 2:

```
> transition%*%priorstate
         [,1]
[1,]  0.995
[2,]  0.005
[3,]  0.000
```

Now we want to update the *currentstate* vector to change values for all subsequent months. We can do that using a "for loop," which says that, for values of time from time point 1 through time point 120, we should update the *currentstate* vector to provide the updated values of p_{non}, p_{rare}, and $p_{routine}$. In R, we do this by type the following code: for (t in 1:timesteps)

This for command tells R to repeat doing something from month 2 until the value of *timesteps*, which is month 120. What should R do? In curved brackets "{}" we can insert a series of commands that R should repeat. Let's tell R to do the following set of commands:

```
for (t in 2:timesteps)
{
 priorstate =c(pnon[t-1],prare[t-1],proutine[t-1])
 newstate= transition%*%priorstate
 pnon[t]=newstate[1]
 prare[t]=newstate[2]
 proutine[t]=newstate[3]
}
```

Here, we see that, within the for loop, we're asking *R* to do three things. First, we're asking it to declare what the prior state is. We create a vector called *priorstate* in which we take the values from the *pnon, prare*, and *proutine* vectors from the prior time period. For example, if *t* is month 2, the *priorstate* vector is constructed using month 1's values. Then we multiply the transition matrix by this *priorstate* vector to get the updated probabilities in the next month. Finally, we tell *R* to assign these new values to the corresponding position in vectors *pnon, prare*, and *proutine*. For example, the value in *newstate* position 3 if *t* is 2 will be the value of *proutine* in month 2.

If we highlight this whole set of code and click "Run," we will produce an output that is equivalent to filling out an entire set of columns in Excel: the vectors *pnon, prare*, and *proutine* will all be filled in for all values of time through month 120. We can check this by typing in the names of the vectors and seeing their updated states at time 120:

```
> pnon[120]
[1] 0.9576078
> prare[120]
[1] 0.03029605
> proutine[120]
[1] 0.01209616
```

As we can see, *pnon* has taken on an eventual steady-state value of about 0.958, while *prare* has taken on a steady state of 0.03 and *proutine* of 0.012, just as we calculated using Excel.

If we want to plot the probability over time of becoming a routine cocaine user, we can just type: plot(proutine) and obtain Figure 7.4. The full *R* code for programming our model in *R* and producing Figure 7.4 is provided on this book's website (https://github.com/sanjaybasu/modelinghealthsystems/).

A COST-EFFECTIVENESS ANALYSIS IN *R*

Now that we have the model programmed in *R*, we can see how powerful *R* can be as opposed to Excel.

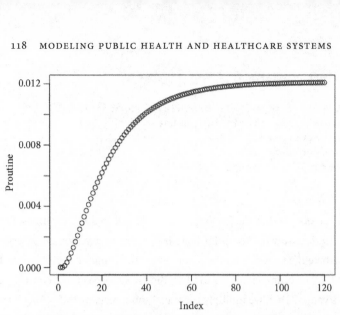

FIGURE 7.4 **Probability over time of becoming a routine cocaine user, based on** *R* **implementation of the Markov model of the Los Angeles cocaine epidemic. "Index" on the x-axis refers to month, and "proutine" on the y-axis to the probability of becoming a routine cocaine user.**

First, suppose we want to simulate 50 years instead of just 10 years of time. In Excel, this task would require us to simulate the model for 50*12 = 600 rows, whereas in R we just have to change one variable: *timesteps* = 600. Despite the long time for the modeling, the simulation should still run in less than a second. R is much more capable of doing large-scale computations rapidly and efficiently. For most modern Markov models, we are not limited to three states of disease, but instead have numerous states and complex transitions and are called upon to simulate the entire lifetime of individuals (often up to 100 years of age). Hence, R becomes much more computationally efficient than Excel to use for most Markov models.

Second, R can help us conduct a cost-effectiveness analysis rapidly. We can recall from Chapter 5 that an intervention for preventing the use of cocaine changed our transition matrix to the following equation:

$$\begin{bmatrix} 0.9975 & 0.15 & 0.02 \\ 0.0025 & 0.826 & 0.04 \\ 0 & 0.024 & 0.94 \end{bmatrix} \begin{bmatrix} p_{non}(t-1) \\ p_{rare}(t-1) \\ p_{routine}(t-1) \end{bmatrix} = \begin{bmatrix} p_{non}(t) \\ p_{rare}(t) \\ p_{routine}(t) \end{bmatrix}. \qquad \text{[Equation 7.3]}$$

We can create a copy of the code from which to calculate the new outcomes given the new transition matrix. We can just cut and paste our R code and label the new transition matrix and new probabilities with "_prev" to distinguish them from our baseline simulation:

```
transition_prev = matrix(c(0.9975,0.15,0.02,0.0025,0.826,0.04
,0,0.024,0.94),ncol=3,byrow=TRUE)
```

```
pnon_prev = rep(0,timesteps)
prare_prev = rep(0,timesteps)
proutine_prev = rep(0,timesteps)
pnon_prev[1]=1
for (t in 2:timesteps)
{
  priorstate_prev =c(pnon_prev[t-1],prare_prev[t-1],proutine_
  prev[t-1])
  newstate_prev= transition_prev%*%priorstate_prev
  pnon_prev[t]=newstate_prev[1]
  prare_prev[t]=newstate_prev[2]
  proutine_prev[t]=newstate_prev[3]
}
pnon_prev[120]
prare_prev[120]
proutine_prev[120]
```

This gives us identical values to what we found in Excel:

```
> pnon_prev[120]
[1] 0.9783461
> prare_prev[120]
[1] 0.0154757
> proutine_prev[120]
[1] 0.006178174
```

Suppose we have the parameters in Table 7.1 for calculating the cost-effectiveness of the intervention.

After running the for loop in *R*, we can calculate costs and QALYs quickly. In a population of 4 million people, costs for the pre-intervention model can be calculated as:

```
costs = sum(4000000*(prare*1+proutine*50)).
```

Table 7.1 Key input assumptions and parameters for a Markov model used to conduct a cost-effectiveness analysis of prevention or treatment for cocaine use

Parameter	Value
Treatment program cost, per routine cocaine user per month	$100
Prevention program cost, per non-user of cocaine per month	$2
Costs generated by each rare cocaine user per month	$1
Costs generated by each routine cocaine user per month	$50
Quality adjusted life-month costs of being a rare user of cocaine per month	0.01
Quality adjusted life-month costs of being a routine user of cocaine per month	0.15

This command first calculates $1 times the probability of being a rare user in a given month, plus $50 times the probability of being a routine user in a given month, multiplied by the population size to get the total costs for Los Angeles, then summed across all months. (If we wanted to include time-discounting, as discussed in Chapter 2, we could divide the expression within the sum() command by 1.03^(1:120/12.) The command divides the vector 1:120 (the month) by the number 12 to get the expression in years, then raises 1.03 to that power, assuming a 3% annual discount rate.

Similarly, costs for the post-intervention model would include the prevention costs:

```
costs_prev = sum(4000000*(prare_prev*1+proutine_prev*50+2*pnon_
prev))
```

Analogously, we could sum QALYs under the pre- and post-intervention conditions:

```
qalys = sum(4000000*(pnon*1+prare*(1-0.01)+proutine*(1-0.15)))/12
qalys_prev = sum(4000000*(pnon_prev*1+prare_prev*(1-0.01)+
proutine_prev*(1-0.15)))/12
```

Here, we've summed the quality-adjusted life-month values and divided by 12 to obtain QALYs. (Again, we can include discounting by dividing each expression within the sum() command by 1.03^(1:120/12)).

Finally, we can compute the incremental cost-effectiveness ratio (ICER) as: (costs_prev-costs)/(qalys_prev-qalys), which gives:

```
> (costs_prev-costs)/(qalys_prev-qalys)
[1] 24076.48
```

Just as we found in Excel, the prevention program costs approximately $24,076 per QALY gained. The full R code for programming our model in R and producing the cost-effectiveness analysis is provided on the book's website.

Unique Flexibilities in *R*: Uncertainty Analysis

So far, we have shown how to reproduce our Markov model from Excel in R, but not clearly indicated anything—except for computational speed—that might convince us that programming in R is uniquely advantageous and provides opportunities we didn't have in Excel.

The first key advantage is to perform *uncertainty analysis*, or the incorporation of uncertain parameters into our models. For example, in our prevention example, we assumed the values in Table 7.1 were the same for everyone in the population. But suppose we have conducted a study and found that the input parameters to our model are not the same for everyone but can vary substantially. Let's take just one parameter for example: the cost of the prevention program. Suppose the cost is $2 per nonuser per month on average, but that the cost can be variable and uncertain because the prevention program makes heavy use of advertising and the cost of advertising is variable and unpredictable. In reality, the cost is $2 per nonuser per month but has a standard deviation of $0.50. Hence, if the cost is normally distributed (Gaussian), the 95% confidence intervals around the $2 estimate are $2 − (1.96 × 0.5) and $2 + (1.96 × 0.5), or from $1.02 to $2.98. This is an incredibly large amount of variation from the perspective of applying the prevention program to 4 million people, among whom a vast majority are nonusers. Hence, we really should know—especially for planning our budget—how much variation we might have in the cost of the program because of the uncertain advertising costs.

How can we incorporate this uncertainty into the Markov model? To our knowledge, there is no way to easily perform this analysis in Excel. But in *R*, we can quickly incorporate the uncertainty in this key parameter and identify how much it might affect our results.

To incorporate uncertainty, we first recognize that *R* can quickly generate random numbers. To generate normally distributed random numbers, we use the rnorm command: `rnorm(n = 10, mean = 2, sd = 0.5)`, and *R* will produce 10 random numbers from a normal distribution with mean 2 and standard deviation 0.5:

```
> rnorm(n = 10, mean = 2, sd = 0.5)
 [1] 1.779351 2.629897 1.236332 1.884404 2.371772
 [6] 1.719896 1.667590 1.584770 2.172189 2.343760
```

We can use the rnorm command to analyze the uncertainty around our cost-effectiveness analysis estimate of the ICER. For example, let's see how much our estimate of the ICER varies if we take into account the uncertainty in advertising dollars.

To conduct such an uncertainty analysis, we should first create a random vector of zeros to fill in for the values of our costs under the prevention program. Just as we created vectors of zeros to fill in for the *pnon*, *prare*, and *proutine* vectors, we can similarly create a vector to fill in for *costs_prev*. Let's say that we want to repeatedly calculate ICER values 10,000 times while sampling repeatedly from the distribution of possible values for the prevention program cost. In other words, we want to find out how much our ICER estimates might vary after we've sampled extensively from the possible values of the prevention program cost. Hence, we can create a vector of zeros for *costs_prev* that is 10,000 numerals long:

```
costs_prev = rep(0,10000)
```

Next, we can create a vector with 10,000 values of the prevention program cost per nonuser person per month; let's call it *prevcost*:

```
prevcos = rnorm(n = 10000, mean = 2, sd = 0.5)
```

Finally, we can make use of the same "for loop" strategy we adopted in programming our Markov model to produce estimates of *costs_prev*:

```
for (val in 1:10000)
{
 costs_prev[val] =sum(4000000*(prare_prev*1+proutine_prev*50+
 prevcost[val]*pnon_prev))
}
```

Here, we are repeating a loop 10,000 times. Within each loop, we are iterating the value of parameter *val* from 1 to 10,000. Our equation for *costs_prev* is identical to its value previously, except that we have replaced the number "2" with the expression *prevcost[val]*, which means that R will sample value number *val* from vector *prevcost*, which is the vector of random normal numbers with mean $2 and standard deviation $0.50. Hence, we are filling in the value of *cost_prev* in position *val* to calculate the cost at each value of the vector *prevcost*.

Once the "for loop" is done, we can recalculate the ICER just as we did earlier:

```
icer = (costs_prev-costs)/(qalys_prev-qalys)
```

This time, however, icer has become a vector of 10,000 values because *costs_prev* had 10,000 values. R smartly kept the other variables the same value when performing the calculation.

How variable is our ICER estimate? We can plot a histogram describing the distribution of the ICER variable by typing the command: hist(icer), which produces Figure 7.5.

As we see in Figure 7.5, there is really wide variability in our ICER estimate due to the seemingly small variability in the $2 per person per month estimate. We can quantify just how wide the variability is by calculating 95% confidence intervals around our estimate by typing quantile(icer, c(0.025, 0.975)). This expression calculates any quantiles of choice, and the vector c(0.025, 0.975) means that we want to calculate the 2.5th percentile and the 97.5th percentile, which corresponds to the 95% confidence intervals:

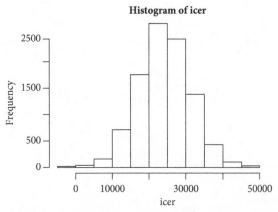

FIGURE 7.5 **A histogram describing the distribution of the incremental cost-effectiveness variable, icer. The x-axis displays values of the icer variable after 10,000 simulations with our model, and the y-axis shows the frequency of values at each icer value.**

```
> quantile(icer, c(0.025,0.975))
    2.5% 97.5%
10667.36 37613.25
```

Hence, our ICER estimate is a mean of $24,076.48, but with a very wide 95% confidence interval, from $10,667.36 to $37,613.25.

We can add further uncertainty analyses by following the preceding protocol and can even account for the uncertainty in multiple variables at once using this procedure to get a better sense of what level of confidence we might have in our model estimates.

In the next few chapters, we'll learn more about the power of using *R* to create models that are difficult or impossible to create using spreadsheets, and we'll see how we can further incorporate uncertainty analysis and related forms of probabilistic thinking into our analyses.

8

MICROSIMULATION

In previous chapters, we used Markov models to estimate the burden of disease and the potential impact of our interventions. One of the key limitations to Markov models is that they don't take into account a person's unique individual characteristics: Markov models are designed to efficiently simulate the average outcome for an entire population. For many public health and healthcare system problems, however, we need to consider *heterogeneity* within a population, or differences in risk and benefit from our programs. For that purpose, *microsimulation* models, which take into account unique characteristics of individuals and the correlations between these characteristics, can be more useful. In this chapter, we detail the construction and use of microsimulation models, using examples related to diabetes prevention and treatment.

SCREENING FOR TYPE 2 DIABETES

In 2013, Dr. Akihiro Seita of the United Nations' Relief and Works Agency (UNRWA) sent out an email to diabetes experts around the world. Dr. Seita was in charge of a massive UN system of hospitals and clinics that care for refugees in the Middle East. In total, he oversaw 3,000 staff at 138 hospitals and clinics serving 5 million refugees.

Although Dr. Seita had dealt with numerous complex problems—clean water delivery, transportation problems in conflict zones, and infectious disease outbreaks—he had recently encountered a problem he hadn't anticipated: the rising prevalence of type 2 diabetes among refugees.

In his email to diabetes experts. Dr. Seita explained that numerous refugees were coming to hospitals and clinics with complications of diabetes, such as blindness, stroke, and kidney failure. It was thought that the prevalence of the disease might be as high as 1 in 5 adults, but few people were diagnosed in time to avoid the complications of the illness. The refugees' diet might have been part of the issue because humanitarian food packages were often loaded with carbohydrates.

In response to his email, Dr. Seita received dozens of suggestions about what to do. Most of the experts suggested screening people in the community for diabetes. Some experts thought Dr. Seita should widely administer a blood test for diabetes, which is a fasting (early morning, before eating) blood sugar test. Those people with fasting blood sugar levels of 126 mg/dL or higher are said to have diabetes. But Dr. Seita's budget was so limited that he couldn't administer many blood tests. He needed a survey that could be cheaply administered to a large population of people to find those at highest risk for diabetes; those at high risk, according to the survey, could be sent to health clinics to get a blood test.

Finding a survey to screen for diabetes risk was not a problem; there were dozens of surveys available. The question was which survey might best serve Dr. Seita's population. Different surveys used different criteria to determine who was considered "high risk" for diabetes. One survey suggested that everyone with a waist circumference greater than 80 centimeters should be considered "high risk." Another survey suggested that a combination of two factors would be necessary to be considered "high risk": a waist circumference greater than 80 centimeters and a systolic blood pressure reading of at least 140 mm Hg. Yet a third survey suggested that only those people with a systolic blood pressure reading of at least 150 mm Hg and with a body mass index (BMI) of at least 30 kg/m² should be considered "high risk," regardless of their waist circumference.

Which screening instrument should Dr. Seita choose? Dr. Seita ultimately wanted to use whichever screening tool let him find the most people with diabetes (a highly sensitive test) with the fewest false-positive screening test results (a highly specific test). The goal was to detect people with diabetes in time to give them treatment and avoid complications of the disease.

THE MOTIVATION FOR MICROSIMULATION

Suppose that we wanted to answer Dr. Seita's question using a Markov model. A typical Markov model of type 2 diabetes might have just two states: a healthy state for people without diabetes and a state for people with diabetes (Figure 8.1). The flow

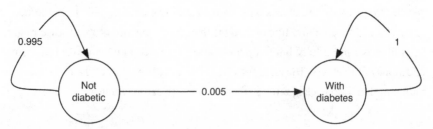

FIGURE 8.1 Markov model of type 2 diabetes.

between the two states would be the rate of diabetes in the population. But how would we be able to use such a model to compare the screening tools? The model would only have the average rate of diabetes in the population. Those people with diabetes would be the group that the screening surveys should find; the more of these people who screen positive, the more sensitive the test. The fewer people who are healthy who screen positive, the more specific the test. But how do we know which subset of people within each state would test positive? The Markov model, as drawn in Figure 8.1, can't tell us anything about individual features of the people in each state: it just lumps all people together based on whether they are healthy or have diabetes.

If we wanted to use the Markov model to capture how different screening tools might work in the refugee population, perhaps one strategy would be to break up each of the states into different populations of people: those with a large waist circumference, those with high blood pressure, and those with high BMI, for example. Such a model is shown in Figure 8.2. As shown here, we can now try to estimate

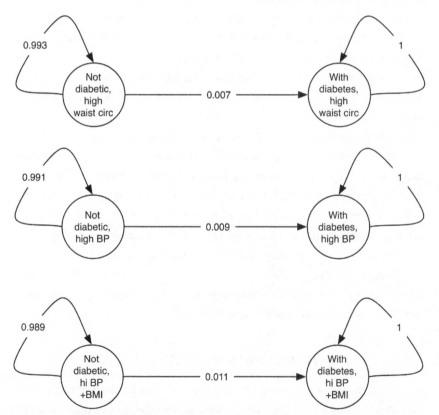

FIGURE 8.2 Markov models of type 2 diabetes, in which each of the states are subdivided into different populations of people: those with a large waist circumference, those with high blood pressure, and those with high body mass index.

what the rate of diabetes is among people with a large waist circumference, what the rate of diabetes is among people with high blood pressure, and what the rate of diabetes is among people with high ##BMI. Figure 8.2 shows some typical rates from Dr. Seita's population. One screening survey would people with high waist circumference. Another would affect people with high waist circumference and high blood pressure. A third instrument would affect the people with a different definition of high blood pressure, and high BMI.

Despite making our Markov model more complex, we still face major problems with utilizing it to identify the best screening instrument: there will be people who fall simultaneously into many of these states. For example, some people will have all three risk factors (high waist circumference, high blood pressure, and high BMI). Presumably, these people will be at the highest risk for diabetes. Other people will have two of the three, and some people will have just one risk factor or no risk factors. Also, it's unclear how we should define "high blood pressure" when it's a continuous measure, and one instrument uses a cutoff of 140 mm Hg to define "high blood pressure" while another uses a cutoff of 150 mm Hg.

A natural next step is to try to make a Markov model that has states for every possible combination of features: a state for people with just high waist circumference, or both high waist circumference and high blood pressure, or with various combinations of states that can account for both definitions of high blood pressure. Very quickly, we would have a large number of different states and an unmanageably complex model.

The natural alternative to making such a complex model would be to ultimately make enough states that we can capture every combination of characteristics we would want to simulate. We can reduce the model all the way from the broad population to each individual, taking into account each individual's unique risk factors within the population. A model that takes into account the unique properties of each individual is known as a *microsimulation*. Rather than just describing a group of people and what state they are in (a Markov modeling approach), a microsimulation is like a large table describing each person in the population. As demonstrated in Table 8.1, an individual in the table may have one or more risk factors, and all 5 million people might be considered in the model.

CONSTRUCTING A MICROSIMULATION

To construct a microsimulation, there are two tools that we need: (1) an estimate of the distributions of characteristics we want to simulate (such as their means and standard deviations) and (2) an estimate of how correlated those characteristics are.

Table 8.1 Tabular conceptualization of a microsimulation

Person number	Waist Circumference (cm)	Blood Pressure (mm Hg)	Body Mass Index (kg/m²)	Fasting Blood Sugar (mg/dL)
1	48	128	17	138
2	86	136	28	110
3	92	159	32	173
4	68	135	25	91
...				
5,000,000	81	139	30	123

Dr. Seita provided us with these estimates: in a brief survey of a subsample of his refugee population, people had a mean waist circumference of 75 cm (standard deviation [SD] = 10 cm), a mean blood pressure of 130 mm Hg (SD = 25 mm Hg), a mean BMI of 25 kg/m² (SD = 5 kg/m²), and a fasting blood sugar of 108 mg/dL (SD = 20 mg/dL). Table 8.2 shows the correlation among these characteristics as a *correlation matrix*, which is a set of Pearson correlation coefficients capturing the relationship between each factor and every other factor (the coefficient captures how often each set of factors is found commonly with each other set of factors; i.e., higher waist circumferences are positively correlated with having higher blood pressure, which is positively correlated with having higher BMI, which is positively correlated with higher fasting blood sugars).

It's important to take into account the correlation between factors because our screening survey instruments are trying to capture the highest risk people who presumably have two or three of the risk factors of high waist circumference, high blood pressure, or high BMI.

Table 8.2 Correlation matrix of type 2 diabetes risk factors in a refugee population

	Waist Circumference (cm)	Blood Pressure (mm Hg)	Body Mass Index (kg/m²)	Fasting Blood Sugar (mg/dL)
Waist circumference	1.000	0.302	0.571	0.776
High blood pressure	0.302	1.000	0.110	0.587
Body mass index	0.571	0.110	1.000	0.002
Fasting blood sugar	0.776	0.587	0.002	1.000

Next, we need to turn on *RStudio* (see Chapter 7) and use our two pieces of information—the distribution (mean and standard deviation) of each characteristic and the correlation among characteristics—to construct a simulated refugee population.

To construct our population, we open a new code window and insert the input parameters we need to provide this population with the key characteristics for each individual. This example will illustrate the power of *R*: there is no way, to our knowledge, to construct such a microsimulation in Excel. The full code for the subsequent microsimulation is also available for download on this book's website (https://github.com/sanjaybasu/modelinghealthsystems/).

In our code, first let's declare the sample size we want to simulate:

```
n = 5000000
```

Here, variable *n* is being given a value of 5 million, the number of people we want to simulate.

Next, we need to input the prevalence and standard deviation (uncertainty around the prevalence) of each of the four characteristics we're trying to include in our simulation: high waist circumference, family history, high blood pressure, and fasting blood sugar. Let's create a vector of prevalence of characteristics and another vector of standard deviations around those prevalence estimates:

```
chars=c(75, 130, 25, 108)
sds=c(10, 25, 5, 20)
```

Here, we have the characteristics in the order stated: waist circumference, blood pressure, BMI, and blood sugar. Our next step is to insert our correlation matrix:

```
cormat = matrix(c(1.000,0.302, 0.571, 0.776,
                  0.302, 1.000, 0.110, 0.587,
                  0.571, 0.110, 1.000, 0.002,
                  0.776,0.587, 0.002, 1.000),ncol=4,byrow=TRUE)
```

Just as described in Chapter 7, we have a matrix with four columns, read row by row from left to right.

The critical next step is to use these two pieces of information—distribution of characteristics and correlation between them—to generate a simulated population. To do this, we need to make use of a key feature of *R*: the ability to install packages that external users have created to save us time and do tasks that are not built in to *R* by default. Installing packages is like installing apps on a smartphone or adding a turbo drive to a car engine—they help us do new things and can rapidly expand our capabilities. We'll install two packages for microsimulation by typing in the following commands:

```
install.packages('MASS')
install.packages('MBESS')
library(MASS)
library(MBESS)
```

The first two lines (install.packages) only have to be run once; the packages are then installed on your hard drive and don't need to be run again. The next two lines (library) tell *R* to activate the packages, just like clicking and starting an app on a smartphone. They need to be run every time we start up the program.

Now that the two packages are installed and activated, we can use them. We first want to create a table similar to Table 8.1, in which the prevalence rates and correlations between characteristics in the refugee population can be translated into a simulation of people and their unique characteristics. We will need to convert the correlation matrix into a *covariance matrix*, which is simply a translation of correlation statistics into a scaled and standardized format; the covariance reflects how much the factors vary together, taking into account their standard deviations, and can be calculated from the correlation matrix using the MBESS package in *R*:

```
sigma=cor2cov(cormat,sds)
```

Here, we use the cor2cov function in the MBESS package to convert the correlation matrix to a covariance matrix.

Next, we take into account both the prevalence and the covariance matrix to simulate a population of 5 million people. We create a sample of characteristics that simultaneously matches the distribution of each individual characteristic in the population (its mean and standard deviation) and the correlation between characteristics in the population (the correlation matrix). To do so, we use the MASS package in *R*:

```
pop=mvrnorm(n,chars,sigma)
```

We specifically create a new matrix *pop* using the mvrnorm function in the MASS package, which takes the number of samples we want (n = 5 million), the means (*chars* vector), and the covariance matrix (*sigma* matrix) and—after a moment of computation—produces a table of 5 million people and their characteristics that is similar to Table 8.1. The function creates a multivariate (many variables) normal distribution of each characteristic to match the distribution and covariance matrix for the population. If non-normal or other atypical distributions are called for, the Help function in *RStudio* provides a guide to sampling from many other types of distributions.

Once we have created our matrix of people, we can examine it. We might not want to view the whole table at once, since it's 5 million rows long for the 5 million people we have simulated. We can see the first 10 rows by using the *R* command head:

```
> head(pop, 10)
           [,1]      [,2]      [,3]      [,4]
 [1,] 71.94014 114.0875 26.52497  92.55315
 [2,] 64.61419 121.3492 18.49197 100.20444
 [3,] 74.93484 163.1153 26.97546 110.30267
 [4,] 81.88704 145.4949 30.98941 112.00721
 [5,] 87.48825 146.8071 21.51043 146.29444
 [6,] 82.96516 144.4435 33.76540 106.99635
 [7,] 70.59627 131.9912 25.55418  97.47015
 [8,] 71.65715 118.3817 20.14378 109.57800
 [9,] 90.48061 143.9922 30.41948 128.85458
[10,] 85.66734 165.6580 34.77085 115.84608
```

We see that, in column 1, we have a series of waist circumference values; in column 2, we have a series of blood pressure values; in column 3, we have a series of body mass indices; and in column 4, we have fasting blood sugar values.

Of course, because we're doing a simulation with random numbers, the exact numbers will change from simulation to simulation. But what we hope to achieve is to fairly compare our screening instruments in a simulated large population such that, on average, we will get the correct means, distributions, and correlations as in the real population (per the Central Limit Theorem of statistics). By simulating a large population, we can hope to identify how certain or uncertain we are about the comparisons among the three screening instruments. We can even perform the whole simulation multiple times (as we did in Chapter 7) to capture variations in our outcome based on uncertainty in our input parameter values.

How do we know that our simulation has correctly captured the distribution of characteristics in our population and the correlation between characteristics? We can use a few commands to ensure that our simulation has matched our two key pieces of information:

```
install.packages('matrixStats')
library(matrixStats)
colMeans(pop)
colSds(pop)
cor(pop)
```

Here, we installed a package called *matrixStats*, which allows us to quickly calculate statistics on matrices. We then activated the package using the `library` command and then checked that the means, standard deviations, and correlation matrix of our resulting matrix *pop* corresponded well to our input data. The `col-Means` command takes the means of each column of the matrix, the `colSds` command takes the standard deviations of each column, and the `cor` command gives us the correlation matrix.

We can even plot the values of characteristics and visualize their correlation:

```
pairs(~pop[1:1000,1]+pop[1:1000,2]+pop[1:1000,3]+
pop[1:1000,4])
```

Whenever calling elements of a matrix in R, square brackets tell R which row and which column to refer to; so [1,2] means row 1, column 2, while [2,] means row 2, all columns, and [,3] means all rows for column 3. Hence, in the preceding command, we've asked R to plot all pairs of values for the first 1,000 rows of each column against each other; we only chose to plot 1,000 values because 5 million values take a lot of processing power and can't be easily visualized. The resulting plot is shown in Figure 8.3.

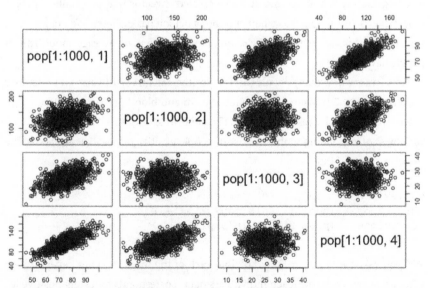

FIGURE 8.3 Scatter plot of pairs of values for the first 1,000 rows of each column against each other, in the microsimulation of type 2 diabetes screening. Pop[1:1000,1] refers to rows 1 through 1000, column 1 (the waist circumference). Similarly, column 2 corresponds to systolic blood pressure, column 3 to body mass index, and column 4 to fasting blood glucose. The x and y axes display values of each variable against each other.

USING THE MICROSIMULATION
TO COMPARE INTERVENTIONS

Now that we have constructed our simulated population, we can use it to compare our three diabetes screening survey instruments.

One survey suggested that everyone with a waist circumference greater than 80 centimeters should be considered "high risk." A second survey suggested that a combination of two factors would be necessary to be considered "high risk": a waist circumference greater than 80 centimeters and a systolic blood pressure of at least 140 mm Hg. Yet a third survey suggested that only those people with a blood pressure of at least 150 mm Hg and with a BMI of at least 30 kg/m² should be considered "high risk," regardless of their waist circumference.

Suppose that we wanted to find the instrument with the highest sensitivity and highest specificity for finding people with diabetes.

First, we need to convert the fasting blood sugar values into a dichotomous variable for whether or not a person has diabetes:

```
dm = (pop[,4]>=126)
```

Here, we ask R whether the value in column 4 of the *pop* matrix is greater than or equal to 126 mg/dL; if so, R returns a value of 1, and otherwise returns a value of 0. Using the preceding command, we've created a vector that is 5 million people long, with 0's and 1's to tell us whether or not a person has diabetes. We can get some statistics on this variable by typing mean(dm) to see that, on average about, 18% of people have diabetes.

Now let's see how many people will test positive for survey 1 (waist circumference >80 cm), survey 2 (waist circumference >80 cm and blood pressure ≥140 mm Hg), and survey 3 (blood pressure ≥150 mm Hg and BMI ≥30 kg/m²). We can create three variables corresponding to the number of people positive or negative on each of the three surveys:

```
survey1pos = (pop[,1]>80)
survey2pos = (pop[,1]>80)&(pop[,2]>=140)
survey3pos = (pop[,2]>=150)&(pop[,3]>=30)
```

We have asked R to put in 1's and 0's into each of the three variables depending on whether or not each row (each individual's data) corresponds to testing positive for each screening test. Notice that R allows us to rapidly process the entire 5-million-person-long row of data in just one command.

We can quickly tabulate how many people tested positive with each survey tool by using the `table` command:

```
> table(survey1pos)
survey1pos
  FALSE    TRUE
3457967 1542033
> table(survey2pos)
survey2pos
  FALSE    TRUE
4265047  734953
> table(survey3pos)
survey3pos
  FALSE    TRUE
4790793  209207
```

If we want to see what percentage tested positive, we just have to divide by the total population size, n:

```
> table(survey1pos)/n
survey1pos
     FALSE      TRUE
0.6915934 0.3084066
> table(survey2pos)/n
survey2pos
     FALSE      TRUE
0.8530094 0.1469906
> table(survey3pos)/n
survey3pos
     FALSE      TRUE
0.9581586 0.0418414
```

Finally, we can calculate the sensitivity and specificity of each survey instrument. The sensitivity is the number of people testing positive divided by all people with the condition, whereas the specificity is the number testing negative divided by all people without the condition.

The sensitivity can be translated into *R* code as:

```
sens1 = sum(((survey1pos==1)&(dm==1)))/sum(dm==1)
sens2 = sum(((survey2pos==1)&(dm==1)))/sum(dm==1)
sens3 = sum(((survey3pos==1)&(dm==1)))/sum(dm==1)
```

Here, we determine the total (sum) number of people who are both positive in testing by a survey instrument and have diabetes, divided by the total testing positive.

Analogously, the specificity can be coded as:

```
spec1 = sum(((survey1pos==0)&(dm==0)))/sum(dm==0)
spec2 = sum(((survey2pos==0)&(dm==0)))/sum(dm==0)
spec3 = sum(((survey3pos==0)&(dm==0)))/sum(dm==0)
```

Comparing the outcomes, we see that the sensitivities and specificities are:

```
> sens1
[1] 0.8050339
> sens2
[1] 0.5482468
> sens3
[1] 0.09512384
> spec1
[1] 0.8037088
> spec2
[1] 0.9433038
> spec3
[1] 0.9704223
```

We see that, overall, survey instrument 1 is best from the perspective of maximizing sensitivity (at 81% sensitivity), and it has 80% specificity as well. Survey instrument 2 is unimpressive in terms of sensitivity (55%), but has higher specificity (94%). Survey instrument 3 has terrible sensitivity (only 10% sensitivity), but is best from the perspective of preventing false positives (specificity 97%).

Ultimately, none of the three instruments is very impressive, but we could use our model to test alternative instruments using combinations of instruments to improve performance. One common way that epidemiologists compare the performance statistics of tests is to plot a *receiver operating characteristic* (ROC) curve. The ROC curve plots 1 minus the specificity of an instrument against the sensitivity of an instrument, and a *C-statistic* is calculated as the area under the curve. Higher *C*-statistics (closer to 1) indicate a better ability of an instrument to discriminate people with the disease from those without.

We can use the Epi package in *R* to calculate the *C* statistic:

```
install.packages('Epi')
library(Epi)
ROC(survey1pos, dm)
```

The ROC function requires us to first type the test results, then the true disease status, in parentheses. The ROC curve for instrument 1 is shown in Figure 8.4, which reveals a *C*-statistic of 0.804. Typically, we aim for *C*-statistics that are higher than

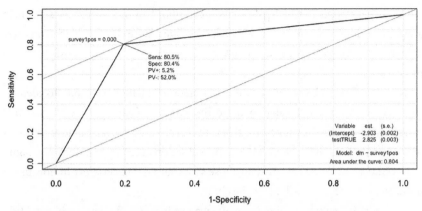

FIGURE 8.4 We compare the performance statistics of survey instrument #1 by plotting a "receiver operating characteristic" (ROC) curve. The ROC curve plots 1 minus the specificity of an instrument against the sensitivity of an instrument, and a *C-statistic* is calculated as the area under the curve. Higher *C-statistics* (closer to 1) indicate a better ability of an instrument to discriminate people with the disease from those without.

0.8 for an instrument to be considered strong, but for screening purposes we would favor a high-sensitivity instrument over a high-specificity instrument to detect as many people as possible who have the disease.

Addressing Decision Uncertainties Using Microsimulation

Our previous example of microsimulation permitted us to examine how microsimulation can help us detect individuals at different degrees of risk for an outcome, overcoming a hurdle of Markov modeling that tends to focus on the population average rate of disease.

Another important advantage of microsimulation is its ability to allow us to make better decisions when we face a lot of uncertainty. Let's take the following example: suppose we have a medical clinic for which we need to make a hiring decision. Can we afford to hire a new nurse to help us at the clinic?

Currently, we have five doctors at the clinic who see on average 110 patients per day among them (standard deviation of 15), for every day of the 240 days per year that the clinic is open. Because different patients have different levels of illness, they take different amounts of time. Furthermore, because different patients have different insurance companies and require different levels of service, the clinic gets paid different amounts per patient, with the typical patient visit producing $100 in gross revenue (standard deviation of $20). Suppose the clinic currently employs a number of nurses, medical assistants, and receptionists, as well as paying for rent, equipment, and utilities. In total, each year, the collective salary and overhead costs at the clinic total about $2,600,000.

The key question is whether the clinic can afford to hire a new nurse to help around the clinic. The nurse can help make the clinic more efficient so that, on average, another five patients per day might be seen. But the nurse also costs $100,000 in salary.

To solve this problem, we can use our microsimulation methods to identify whether the clinic may be able to afford the expense of hiring a new nurse while taking into account the numerous uncertainties along the way: the uncertainty in how many patients the doctors at the clinic will see on different days, the uncertainty in how much the clinic gets paid for those visits, and the uncertainty in how much more efficient the nurse will make the clinic.

Let's start by putting in the data we have available for the base case condition (before hiring an additional nurse), starting with the number of days the clinic is open:

```
daysperyr = 240
```

We can then estimate the typical visits per year at the clinic, which can be simulated by sampling the number of visits per day (mean = 110, SD = 15) for each of the 210 days per year:

```
visitsperyr = rnorm(n=daysperyr,mean=110,sd=15)
```

Next, we calculate the total gross revenues at the clinic by sampling from the revenue per visit (mean = $100, SD = $20), for each of the visits per year at the clinic:

```
revpervisit = rnorm(n=visitsperyr,mean=100, sd=20)
```

Finally, we add up the total expected gross revenue for the clinic per year:

```
grossrev = sum(visitsperyr*revpervisit)
```

We can determine the current net, after subtracting $2,600,000 in salary and overhead costs from our gross revenue:

```
netrev = (annualrev-2600000)
```

Next, we repeat the process after taking into account the increased revenue from adding our nurse, which is derived from adding another 5 patients per day and subtracting the additional $100,000 in salary:

```
visitsperyr = rnorm(n=daysperyr,mean=110+5,sd=15)
revpervisit = rnorm(n=visitsperyr,mean=100, sd=20)
grossrev = sum(visitsperyr*revpervisit)
netrev = (annualrev-2600000)-100000
```

The variable *netrev* tells us how much money is left over if we hired the additional nurse; it will be positive if we can afford the nurse and negative otherwise. As shown here, we just sample one time for one year's worth of simulated visits and revenues. We want to determine how often we might be able to safely hire a nurse, so we should repeatedly sample from the distributions of uncertainty to determine how often the *netrev* result is a positive number.

We can choose an arbitrarily large number of times (let's say 100,000) to repeat the entire simulation and plot how many times we get a positive revenue outcome. One way to do that is to create an empty vector of zeros to store our results from each of the 1 million simulations and then fill in the results using a "for loop" as in Chapter 7:

```
revresults=rep(0,100000)
for (i in 1:100000){
 daysperyr = 240
 visitsperyr = rnorm(n=daysperyr,mean=110+5,sd=15)
 revpervisit = rnorm(n=visitsperyr,mean=100, sd=20)
 grossrev = sum(visitsperyr*revpervisit)
 netrev = (grossrev-2600000)-100000
revresults[i] = netrev
}
```

Finally, we can plot the results as a histogram, as shown in Figure 8.5.

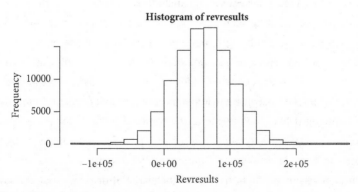

FIGURE 8.5 **Histogram of net revenues after hiring a new nurse at a clinic, using microsimulation.** The x-axis shows the 'revresults' variable corresponding to net annual revenue at the clinic, and the y-axis shows the frequency of each value for net revenue across 100,000 repeated simulations. As shown, most but not all simulations resulted in a positive net revenue after the new nurse was hired.

We can see that we're not 100% certain that we'll always have a positive revenue outcome. What proportion of the time did we end up with a positive result? We can tabulate the percent of the time that our result was positive:

```
> table(revresults>0)/100000

  FALSE    TRUE
0.08058 0.91942
```

It looks like about 92% of the time, of our 100,000 simulations, the clinic was able to afford the nurse.

This example shows how we can use *R*'s ability to perform repeated large-scale simulations and repeated sampling from probability distributions to track uncertainty in a decision and get a sense of whether the decision might be wise or not. In most circumstances, we don't have definite confidence that our mean results are reflective of what will happen every day, month, or year. In uncertain contexts, *R* can help us plan our budgets and resource allocations with a better appreciation for the risks and benefits we might experience.

Agent-Based Modeling: An Extension of Microsimulation

An increasingly popular extension of microsimulation is known as *agent-based modeling*. Agent-based models simulate individuals but have a critical feature that standard microsimulation models do not: they include equations to describe the *behavior* of individuals, not just their fixed features like waist circumference or BMI. For example, an agent-based model of type 2 diabetes might incorporate how much a person drinks sugary beverages and include equations to describe how much higher the risk of drinking such beverages might be if a person is surrounded by other people who also drink sugary beverages (e.g., social contagion).

To extend our diabetes example, we can move from the Middle East to the other side of the world—to the country of Mexico—where behavioral responses to diabetes risk factors have become a major subject of national concern. In recent years, the epidemiologist Juan Dommarco at the National Institute for Public Health in Mexico studied strategies to reduce the risk of type 2 diabetes among young people drinking sugary soda drinks. Dr. Dommarco was asked to estimate what impact the central government might have on diabetes risk if drinking soda did not continue to increase in popularity but was substituted with clean drinking water and was made less popular through marketing campaigns and taxes on soda imposed by the government.

This book's website links to R code that describes an agent-based model of sugary soda consumption. The model of drink consumption has features common to many agent-based models. It can be constructed much like a microsimulation, but with an extra step: in addition to simulating the population and assigning fixed attributes to that population, we additionally set behavioral "decision rules" that describe how people act and interact with each other. Individuals decide, in our case, whether to drink soda based in part on how many others around them are drinking soda.

We use a classical equation for simulating product consumption in a population over time (called the *Bass diffusion model*; note that we present a version of the model commonly used in public health, although numerous other versions also exist with additional complexities).[1] The model can be described by Equation 8.1:

$$\frac{dP(t)}{dt} = \frac{q}{m} P(t) \big[m - P(t) \big].$$ [Equation 8.1]

In Equation 8.1, $P(t)$ is the average probability that a person consumes soda in year t, m is the typical maximum fraction of the population that will be willing to consume soda at some point, and q is a "social diffusion" parameter describing how easily a person is influenced to consume soda by their peers. Based on fitting the model to data from Mexico, we found typical values for the parameters q and m for the population in Mexico, which are inserted into the R code ($q = 0.1159$, $m = 1$). The intuition behind the model formula is that the change in the probability of consuming soda is proportional to some degree of social influence q, as well as a logistic curve (Figure 8.6), such that consumption becomes popular initially and then slows in popularity as the probability of consumption reaches the maximum consumption level m in the population.

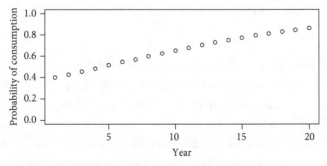

FIGURE 8.6 In an agent-based model of soda consumption, soda consumption becomes popular initially and then slows in popularity as the probability of consumption reaches a maximum consumption level.

To create the model, we first begin by specifying our parameters:

```
n=100000
q=0.1159
m=1
rr=1.4
dmrisk=0.01
p=0.4
time=20
```

Here, we are simulating a representative 100,000 people (*n*) with a given set of social diffusion parameters. We also specify that drinking soda confers a relative risk (*rr*) of diabetes of 1.4 as compared to people not drinking soda and that the baseline (non–soda-drinker) risk of diabetes each year is 0.01 (1%). We specify that the starting probability of drinking soda is 40% (*p*), and we want to simulate a 20-year time period.

Next, we create vectors that use the binomial probability function (rbinom) to determine whether people at the beginning of the model are drinking soda or not and whether people have diabetes or not. The binomial probability function acts like a weighted coin, where the chances of flipping to "heads" (which means the person will consume soda or has diabetes) is given by a probability. The function rbinom creates a vector of length *n*, flipping a coin once per each person, with probability *p* of drinking soda (or 0.15 of having diabetes):

```
soda = rbinom(n,1,p)
dm = rbinom(n,1,0.15)
```

We have to create some vectors to keep track of the total number of soda drinkers and diabetes cases over time:

```
totsoda = sum(soda)
totdm = sum(dm)
```

We then simulate the rate of diabetes conditional on whether someone drinks soda, taking into account the higher rate of diabetes among people who are soda drinkers. Specifically, at each time step of our "for loop" from time point 2 to 20, we will first calculate the probability of soda consumption. We then create the vector *soda* by sampling from a binomial probability function to determine whether people that year are drinking soda or not. We create vector *newdm* to then simulate their risk of diabetes, taking into account the relative risk of diabetes if drinking soda. Finally, we update our vector *dm* to account for new diabetes cases. Note that because diabetes is irreversible, we only update the subset of cases that don't yet have diabetes (dm==0)*newdm. We keep track of the total soda consumers and total cases of diabetes in our vectors *totsoda* and *totdm*:

```
for (i in 2:time){
   p[i] = p[i-1] + (q/m)*p[i-1]*(m-p[i-1])
   soda = rbinom(n,1,p[i])
   newdm = rbinom(n,1,dmrisk*rr*soda)
   dm = (dm==1)+(dm==0)*newdm
   totsoda = c(totsoda,sum(soda))
 totdm = c(totdm, sum(dm))
}
```

We see that the viral social phenomenon of drinking soda could dramatically increase the prevalence of diabetes over the simulated period:

```
> totdm
[1] 15055 15551 16086 16646 17243 17867 18532 19226 19922 20651
21450 22256 23031
[14] 23822 24596 25494 26372 27259 28087 28942
```

By including a "decision rule" in which people drink soda conditional on its popularity, we can simulate how much government intervention would have to change the maximum number of people willing to consume soda (parameter *m*) to affect diabetes rates. In our model, we find that even changes to the number of people willing to consume soda may produce modest changes in diabetes rates, even over very long periods of time. For example, suppose we lowered the parameter *m* from a value of 1 to a value of 0.5 (only half of people are willing to drink soda):

```
> totdm
[1] 14878 15392 15901 16357 16861 17350 17871 18415 18936 19466
19979 20479 20996
[14] 21495 22024 22557 23052 23570 24086 2460
```

By contrast, we can examine how much reducing the social diffusion parameter *q* compares: if we cut *q* in half (from 0.1159 to 0.1159/2), we see that the rates of diabetes are cut to a lesser extent:

```
> totdm
[1] 14819 15324 15866 16392 16919 17496 18032 18578 19145 19743
20376 21000 21619
[14] 22280 22980 23632 24315 24999 25693 26407
```

We could do repeated simulations to compare strategies that affect either or both of these parameters m and q. The simulation can thereby help us estimate the impact of efforts that reduce the influence of peer pressure because preventing just one person from drinking soda may have a multiplicative effect when that individual does not subsequently influence others to drink soda. The multiplicative effect of social influences would have been missed by a traditional microsimulation model—highlighting how an agent-based simulation may assist in revealing phenomena that could not be accounted for if we assumed that a population did not change over time in its disease-relevant features, such as personal behavior.

As shown in this example, both the power and pitfall of agent-based modeling is its complexity: agent-based models can potentially incorporate numerous complexities of how people behave, contingent on the unique circumstances of individuals and the people around them. Yet the "garbage in, garbage out" rule applies—meaning that having good data about people's actual behavioral responses can be critical to implementing an informative agent-based model. Because actual behavioral responses are difficult to identify, researchers often use agent-based modeling for theoretical purposes, such as to identify whether certain kinds of behavioral responses at an individual level produce different results at a population level. For example, in a classical agent-based model of housing segregation in the United States, sociologists found that even if individuals have only slight aversions to living next to people of a race different from themselves, an overall city can become profoundly segregated over time because those small individual biases translate into a very large bias at the population level. This type of finding—in which a population-level phenomena is observed from individual-level behaviors—is known as *emergence*. By revealing emergent phenomena, agent-based models can help to understand why population characteristics (e.g., profound city-level racial segregation) can result from individual characteristics (e.g., only slight racial biases in surveys of racism among individuals).[2]

Another common pitfall of agent-based modeling is to render the behavioral decision rules of simulated people (agents) in the model too complex, such that it is not clear what parameters are producing the overall outcome from the model. For example, our soda consumption model had only two parameters related to the proportion of people willing to consume soda and the speed at which they are influenced by their peers to start consuming soda. However, several other factors may influence an individual's behavior. To clearly define parameters so that independent researchers can replicate the results of an agent-based model, standard international guidelines have been defined (discussed further in Chapter 11),[3] which indicate that researchers should clarify whether a parameter describes "adaptation" (whether and how an individual in the model responds to changes in their properties or properties of their environment), "fitness" (whether and how an individual explicitly calculates how well they are meeting an objective in order to change their behavior, analogous to the concept of fitness in a Darwinian evolutionary sense), "prediction" (whether and how an individual tries to estimate the future consequences of their decision), "sensing" (whether and how an individual senses changes in their properties or properties of their environment, such as how many other people around them are drinking soda), and "interaction" (whether and how an individual interacts with others). By precisely defining behavioral decision rules according to these or similar classification systems, we can hope to understand how different ways of conceptualizing behavior (an inherently complex task) can be scientifically studied to explain real-world phenomena, including risky health behaviors such as tobacco smoking or soda consumption. As with the code in this book, however, the best way to ensure understanding and replication of a model is to share the code producing the model itself.

9

MODELING LARGE-SCALE EPIDEMICS

In previous chapters, we ignored a critical aspect of modeling some major diseases: the infectious nature of many diseases. For infectious diseases, the risk of getting the disease is related to how many people are infectious at a given time: the more infectious people in the area, the higher the risk of infection among susceptible people. In a typical Markov model, we can't account for this basic feature of infectious diseases because the risk of moving from one state (healthy) to another state (diseased) is assumed to be constant. In this chapter, we introduce a simulation modeling framework that has been used for decades to simulate infectious disease epidemics.

USING HAZARD FUNCTIONS

Let's revisit an example we first presented in Chapter 4: the case of a businessperson who is selling marshmallow candies (Peeps) and wants to know how many candies to order from the factory to optimize her profit.

A savvy businessperson could do a simple survey at the Peeps warehouse by asking the warehouse manager, "How long does the average Peep stay on the shelf after it arrives, before it gets ordered and shipped off to the grocery store?" If the answer is 3 days, then what is the average daily per Peep rate of leaving the warehouse? Well, it's 1/3 per day. (That is, 1 Peep/3 days = one-third of a Peep leaving per day). Conversely, if you have a really big fan club of customers, and Peeps fly off your shelf at the rate of 5 per day on average, then what's the average *survival time* of one Peep in your warehouse? It's 1/5 of a day (1 day/5 Peeps = one-fifth of a day on the shelf per Peep).

Therefore, the average survival time of Peeps in your warehouse is:

$$E(T) = \frac{1}{\mu}$$ [Equation 9.1]

where E means the "expectation" (or average) of the time T, which we define as the amount of time a Peep survives on the shelf in your warehouse, and μ is the average per Peep rate of leaving the warehouse.

Let's find a function to describe the probability that a Peep stays on the shelf for at least t units of time. We can write that as $\Pr\{T>t\}$. This is often called a *survival function*, designated $S(t)$. What could this function be? As we first derived in Chapter 4, we can reason that the average shelf life in the warehouse, $E(T)$, is just a sum of 1day*Pr{Peep on shelf 1st day} + 1day*Pr{Peep still on shelf 2nd day} + 1day*Pr{Peep still on shelf 3rd day} + . . . all the way to infinity days (by which time, presumably, the probability of survival has reached 0). In other words,

$$E(T) = \int_0^\infty \Pr\{T > t\}dt = \int_0^\infty S(t)dt = \frac{1}{\mu}. \qquad \text{[Equation 9.2]}$$

We further reasoned in Chapter 4 that a function $S(t)$ that can satisfy this equation, such that its sum from 0 to infinity is $1/\mu$, is the exponential function:

$$\int_0^\infty e^{-\mu t}dt = -\frac{e^{-\mu\times\infty} - e^{-\mu\times0}}{\mu} = -\frac{0-1}{\mu} = \frac{1}{\mu}. \qquad \text{[Equation 9.3]}$$

Hence, we have a function to describe the probability that a Peep survives to time t, shown in Equation 9.4:

$$S(t) = e^{-\mu t}. \qquad \text{[Equation 9.4]}$$

To operationalize this equation, we can reason that if the typical duration of shelf-life for a Peep is 3 days, then the probability that a Peep survives 7 days is $e^{-(1/3)*7} = 0.097$. because 1/3 is the rate of leaving the shelf (1 Peep/3days) and t is 7 days. Hence, there is a 9.7% chance of a Peep surviving a week on the warehouse shelf.

Conversely, we can use Equation 9.4 to convert from a metric of time to a probability of survival. For example, suppose we want to know how much time it would take a Peep's survival probability to be just 25%. We have to solve for t when $S(t) = 0.25$. So $0.25 = e^{-(1/3)*t}$ and, taking the natural logarithm of both sides, we get $ln(0.25) = -(1/3)*t$, which gives $t = 4.2$ days.

How does optimizing our warehouse of Peeps help us to find solutions to stop infectious disease epidemics? We first have to determine how to adjust our equations to address the case of *fluctuating demand*. In other words, if we simulate an infectious disease where the number of people infected per unit time will increase when more people are infectious, we no longer have a constant rate μ but rather have fluctuating rate of infection that could vary widely across time periods. Hence, the survival function—the probability of surviving at least to time t—will not simply be an exponential function of the constant μ summed over all times up to t (i.e., μt), but rather the exponential function of individual rates for each time, $\mu(t)$, summed over all times up to time t:

$$S(t) = e^{-\int_0^t \mu(t)dt}.$$

[Equation 9.5]

The function $\mu(t)$ is commonly referred to as a *hazard function*, meaning the hazardous probability that a Peep will "end its life" at the warehouse (by leaving the warehouse, not via Peep suicide) at a given time t, given that it survived in the warehouse until time t.

Now that we have a survival function that can accommodate a fluctuating rate across time periods, we can convert our model of Peep consumption into a model of infectious disease epidemics.

THE KERMACK-MCKENDRIK MODEL

Suppose we want to conceptualize the process of an epidemic using the classic *Kermack-McKendrick model*, which is also known as the *SIR model* of disease because it has three states that people (a.k.a. "Peeps") can fit into (Figure 9.1). People get shipped around between these states when they are infected with the disease being modeled (moving them from the warehouse of susceptible people to the warehouse of infected people) or recover from infection (moving from the warehouse of infected people to the warehouse of recovered people). The model assumes that the infection is not fatal, that infected people are infectious people, and that recovered people have lifelong immunity. We'll modify the assumptions later in more complex models after we learn the basics. (Note that in some infectious

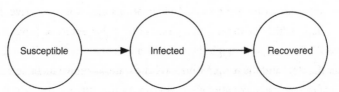

FIGURE 9.1 The classical Kermack-McKendrick "SIR" model depicting infectious disease epidemics in terms of susceptible, infectious, and recovered compartments.

disease literature, states are referred to as *compartments* and the SIR model as a *compartmental model*).

How do we use this simple structure to answer complex questions about controlling infectious disease epidemics? One systematic approach is to label and define all of the rates of flow between states of the model so that we can construct a series of equations to describe the process of infection and recovery.

Based on Equation 9.1, we can reason that the rate of infection can be expressed as the reciprocal of the expected time until a person moves from the susceptible state to the infected state (let's call that $E(T_S)$). The expected time until a person moves from susceptible to infected is the average length of time between birth (which we assume is when a person enters the susceptible state) and the time a person gets infected. Similarly, the rate of recovery can be expressed as the reciprocal of the expected length of time between the infected state and the recovered state; let's call this expected length of time $E(T_I)$.

By this reasoning, if the average age of infection is 10 years, then the average incidence rate of disease per person would be $1/10$ years^{-1}. The average incidence rate per person per unit time is typically called the *force of infection* and is often abbreviated with the Greek letter lambda, λ.

Analogously, if the duration of disease is typically 6 months (0.5 years), then the rate of recovery from the disease per infected person per year is $1/(0.5) = 2$ years^{-1}. Let's call this rate v.

There are two more key rates that haven't been drawn into our diagram but that we'll need to account for in many infectious disease models. One is the birth rate and the other is the death rate. If the population we are simulating is demographically stable—that is, if it's not rising or declining in population size—and the disease is not lethal, then the birth and death rates will be equal. If the average lifetime in the population (let's call it $E(T_L)$) is 75 years, then if we assume an exponential distribution of life expectancy as per Equation 9.1, the rate of death in the population per person would $1/75$ years^{-1}, which in a demographically stable population will also be the rate of birth. We'll call this rate μ.

Now that we have all rates of flow that we need between states, we can write down the equations to describe our model. The equations are easier to derive if we first create a table in which we itemize every rate of flow that enters or leaves each state of our model. We can go through the model state by state to write down the people who enter the state and the people who leave the state, as shown in Table 9.1. For the purposes of the table and equations, we can specify that the susceptible state is letter S, the infected state letter I, and the recovered state letter R. Furthermore, letter N is the total population size (equal to $S + I + R$).

Table 9.1 Equations representing the number of people who enter and leave a given state in the standard Kermack-McKendrick model

State	People Entering State (+)	People Leaving State (−)
Susceptible (S)	Births: birth rate μ per person in population × population size N	Deaths: death rate μ per person in this warehouse × population of this warehouse
		Infections: infection rate λ per susceptible × susceptible population
Infected (I)	Infections: infection rate λ per susceptible × susceptible population	Deaths: death rate μ per person in this warehouse × population of this warehouse
		Recoveries: recovery rate v per infected × infected population
Recovered (R)	Recoveries: recovery rate v per infected × infected population	Deaths: death rate μ per person in this warehouse × population of this warehouse

Translating the table into equation format, we arrive at Equations 9.6 through 9.8, where *t* reflects time:

$$\frac{dS(t)}{dt} = \mu N - \lambda S(t) - \mu S(t) \qquad \text{[Equation 9.6]}$$

$$\frac{dI(t)}{dt} = \lambda S(t) - vI(t) - \mu I(t) \qquad \text{[Equation 9.7]}$$

$$\frac{dR(t)}{dt} = vI(t) - \mu R(t). \qquad \text{[Equation 9.8]}$$

We can quickly check that we have included all of the important rates of disease by adding each of the equations together. Since we have assumed a constant population size, the sum of the right-hand sides of the equations should equal zero, meaning that there is no change in the overall population size. The sum of the right-hand sides equals the expression $\mu * (N - (S + I + R))$, but since $N = (S + I + R)$, the overall expression does in fact add to zero.

As with our Markov models, we can first solve our infectious disease model at a steady state. Under typical steady-state conditions, meaning that the infectious disease roughly infects the same number of people each year, the prevalence of disease is equal to the incidence of disease, multiplied by the duration of disease. To understand this relationship, imagine the analogy of a restaurant: if customers in a restaurant come to eat at a rate of 10 per hour (the incidence of customers) and each stays for 2 hours (the duration of being a customer), then, at any given time, we could reason that the prevalence of customers would be an old batch of 10 customers from the previous hour (who are now in their 2nd hour of eating) and a new batch of 10 from the current hour (who are still in their 1st hour of eating), for a total of 20 customers.

Analogously, we can derive an expression to estimate the steady-state population of infected people in a community. First, we can estimate the prevalence of susceptible people in the stable population. This prevalence will be the "incidence" of being susceptible (i.e., births, μN) multiplied by the "duration" of being in the susceptible state (i.e., the length of time before either dying at rate μ or getting infected at rate λ, which are the only two ways to leave the susceptible state in our model). The expected duration of being in the susceptible state will be $E[\text{minimum}(T_L \text{ or } T_S)]$, since a person will either die first or get infected first, if moving out of the susceptible state. Making use of our survivor function (Equation 9.1):

$$E(\min[T_L, T_S]) = \int_0^\infty e^{-(\mu+\lambda)} dt = \frac{1}{\mu+\lambda}. \qquad \text{[Equation 9.9]}$$

So the number of susceptible people will be the incidence of susceptible people μN times the duration of susceptibility $1/(\mu+\lambda)$, which produces Equation 9.10:

$$S = \frac{\mu N}{\mu+\lambda}. \qquad \text{[Equation 9.10]}$$

Similarly, we can estimate the prevalence of infected people, which will be the incidence of infection (λ times the susceptible population given by equation 9.10) and the duration of infection ($1/(v + \mu)$, by the same logic as above). Hence, the number of infected people will be expressed by Equation 9.11:

$$I = \frac{\mu N}{\mu+\lambda} \times \lambda \times \frac{1}{v+\mu} = \frac{N\mu\lambda}{(\lambda+\mu)(v+\mu)}. \qquad \text{[Equation 9.11]}$$

Equations 9.10 and 9.11 provide us with a useful strategy to estimate prevalence rates for stable diseases in a population that do not wildly fluctuate in incidence each year (*endemic*, rather than epidemic, diseases). For example, if we have a population of 100,000 people with an average life expectancy of 75 years, a force of infection of the disease of interest of 1/10 years^{-1}, and a rate of recovery of 2 years^{-1}, we can calculate the number of susceptible people in the context of this nonfatal, endemic disease at steady state:

$$S = \frac{\mu N}{\mu + \lambda} = \frac{\left(\dfrac{1}{75}\right) \times 100000}{\left(\dfrac{1}{75}\right) + \left(\dfrac{1}{10}\right)} = 11{,}765. \qquad \text{[Equation 9.12]}$$

Around 11,765 people would be expected to remain susceptible to the disease at steady state. Analogously, the number of infected people would be:

$$I = \frac{\mu N}{\mu + \lambda} \times \lambda \times \frac{1}{\nu + \mu} = \frac{N \mu \lambda}{(\lambda + \mu)(\nu + \mu)} = \frac{100000 \times \left(\dfrac{1}{75}\right) \times \left(\dfrac{1}{10}\right)}{\left(\dfrac{1}{10} + \dfrac{1}{75}\right)\left(2 + \dfrac{1}{75}\right)} = 584.$$

[Equation 9.13]

Finally, the number of people who have recovered would be the population size N minus the number of susceptible people, minus the number of infected people, which is 87,651.

THE LAW OF MASS ACTION

While it may be of interest that we can calculate these quantities just using a piece of paper and a pencil, we want to understand how to control diseases that are not at a simple endemic steady-state condition. We must address infectious diseases that are fatal. We can do so by modifying Equations 9.6 through 9.8 by adding an additional rate of death from the infected state to indicate the extra death caused by the disease. This might change the demography of the population if the additional deaths from the disease are not exactly compensated by new births.

Furthermore, we should modify our equations to understand how disease may start out as rare but emerge into an epidemic. How can we account for the fact that, by definition, infectious diseases often do not have constant rates of infection, but rather have changing rates of infection based on the number of infectious people in the population? If there are a lot of infectious people in the population, the risk of infection will be high. If a large number of infectious people are cured of their disease, then the risk of infection will go down.

To solve this problem, we can allude to the challenge we faced when we encountered a changing demand for Peeps: we derived Equation 9.5 to describe how the rate of demand might change over time. Now we can use that equation to describe how the rate of infection can change over time to deal with epidemic diseases for which the infection rate is dynamic.

The most common approach to introduce a dynamic rate of infection is called the *Law of Mass Action*. The Law of Mass Action states that, in a homogeneously mixed population (i.e., a population in which people are circulating around and of generally equivalent risk of being infected with the disease), the incidence rate of the disease will be proportional to the population of infectious people (e.g., the infectious people will be dispersed throughout the community and collide with susceptible people):

$$\lambda(t) = \beta I(t).$$ [Equation 9.14]

For example, suppose that we have a disease for which the force of infection is $1/10$ years^{-1} and the number of people infected currently is 584. We would calculate $\beta = (1/10)/584 = 0.000171$. It is typically the case that β is a small number because it expresses the risk of disease upon one contact between an infectious and a susceptible person per unit time, which should be small.

In Equation 9.14, $\lambda(t)$ is our hazard function for the incidence rate, which changes over time depending on how many infectious $I(t)$ people there are at the time. The constant β is a transmission rate per person per unit time. It tells us how likely it is that a contact between one susceptible person and one infectious person will result in transmission of the disease in question. As a result, it doesn't change for a specific disease in a specific community but instead indicates the "contagiousness" of the specific disease being studied in a particular community.

Using the Law of Mass Action, we can rewrite our series of differential equations (Equations 9.6 – 9.8) by replacing all of the λ's with βI's, to keep track of an epidemic disease whose infection rate changes:

$$\frac{dS(t)}{dt} = \mu N(t) - \beta I(t) S(t) - \mu S(t)$$ [Equation 9.15]

$$\frac{dI(t)}{dt} = \beta I(t) S(t) - v I(t) - \mu I(t)$$ [Equation 9.16]

$$\frac{dR(t)}{dt} = v I(t) - \mu R(t).$$ [Equation 9.17]

Of course, we can still use these equations for an endemic disease at steady state, for which $I(t)$ will be (by definition) constant, such that the force of infection λ will be constant at all times t.

It is common to make some optional modifications to Equation 9.15 through 9.17, particularly by replacing β with two variables multiplied together: the probability of contact between infectious and susceptible people, and the probability that this contact will result in disease transmission. This is useful, for example, when modeling some sexually transmitted diseases, as we will see later in this chapter. Alternatively, it is possible to change λ to equal $\beta I(t)/N$, so that β is multiplied by the fraction of the population that is infectious. The expression scales up the value of β based on the population size.

THE REPRODUCTIVE NUMBER

The *basic reproductive number*, or R_0 (commonly pronounced "are-naught," due to its British origins) is the mean number of secondary infections a single infected person will cause in a population with no immunity to the disease and in the absence of interventions to control the infection. If we imagine an island of people who have never been affected by the disease, then R_0 is the number of people who would be infected by one infected person who lands on the island (a fully susceptible population), before the infected person recovers or dies (is no longer infectious). Figure 9.2 illustrates a disease with an R_0 of 3.

It is important not to confuse R_0 with the *effective reproductive number* (R or R_e, depending on the author), which is the number of secondary cases generated by an infectious case once the epidemic is under way (e.g., once the population is no

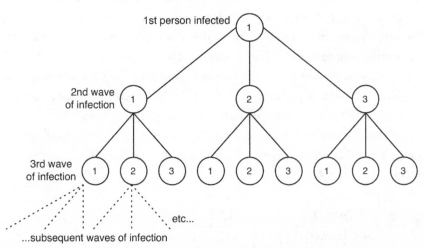

FIGURE 9.2 The basic reproductive number is the number of people in who would be infected by one infected person who lands among a fully-susceptible population, before the infected person recovers or dies (is no longer infectious). The diagram illustrates a disease with a basic reproductive number of three.

longer fully susceptible, but there are some immune persons or some interventions have been introduced such as medical treatment). Of course, we're interested in driving down the effective reproductive number by creating public health programs, but the basic reproductive number is a fundamental property of the disease spread in a given population.

We can reason that if the R_0 of a disease is greater than 1, then one infected person will produce more than one infected person in the next generation of infections on average; hence, the disease will spread. Conversely, if R_0 is less than 1, then one infected person will produce less than one infected person in the next generation of infections on average; hence, the epidemic will eventually burn out.

For epidemic diseases that initially expand, there is some point at which the number of susceptible people will be so few that infected people will not be able to transfer the disease on to as many susceptible people (most people who are in contact with the infected person are either recovered or infected). Hence, the disease transmission process will reach a point when the effective R will be 1, meaning there is some population size S such that:.

$$R_0 \times \frac{S}{N} = 1.$$
[Equation 9.18]

Hence:

$$R_0 = \frac{N}{S}.$$
[Equation 9.19]

The point at which the effective R will be equal to 1 is effectively the point we solved for earlier in the endemic steady-state disease situation, in which the prevalence of being in a given state is equal to the incidence of moving into the state times the duration of being in the state. The "incidence" of being in the population is the birth rate μ times the population that can give birth N, and the "duration" of being in the population is the life expectancy $E(T_L)$. Similarly, the "incidence" of being susceptible is the birth rate μ times the population that can give birth N, and the "duration" of being susceptible is $E[\text{minimum}(T_L \text{ or } T_S)]$, since a person will either die first or get infected first if moving out of the susceptible state. Therefore, Equation 9.19 becomes Equation 9.20:

$$R_0 = \frac{N}{S} = \frac{\mu N E(T_L)}{\mu N E\left[\min(T_L, T_S)\right]} = \frac{E(T_L)}{E\left[\min(T_L, T_S)\right]} \approx \frac{E(T_L)}{E(T_S)} = \frac{\frac{1}{\mu}}{\frac{1}{\mu + \lambda}} = 1 + \frac{\lambda}{\mu}.$$

[Equation 9.20]

The approximation in the midst of this derivation is because T_S is far smaller than T_L in the vast, vast majority of cases (since life expectancy would be longer than the time to get disease).

We can simplify our expression for R_0 further by remembering that $\lambda = \beta I$ and using Equation 9.13:

$$\lambda(t) = \beta I(t) = \frac{\beta N \mu \lambda}{(\lambda + \mu)(v + \mu)}. \qquad \text{[Equation 9.21]}$$

After some simplification and rearrangement, we can substitute Equation 9.21 into Equation 9.20 and end up with this very well-known formula for R_0:

$$R_0 = 1 + \frac{\lambda}{\mu} = \frac{\beta N}{v + \mu} \approx \frac{\beta N}{v}. \qquad \text{[Equation 9.22]}$$

The last approximation is because usually v is much larger than μ.

What we've accomplished here is to use the endemic steady-state expressions to derive a generalizable expression for R_0. This can greatly help us to understand the dangers of a disease and the conditions under which we might be able to control it. For example, suppose we have a population of 100,000 people and a disease for which $\beta = 0.000171$ and $v = 2$ years^{-1}; then, using Equation 9.22, $R_0 = (0.000171*100000)/2 = 8.6$. Each infected person will, on average, infect 8.6 others in a fully susceptible population.

HERD IMMUNITY AND FINAL SIZE CALCULATIONS

Now that we have completed some considerable algebra to derive estimates of steady-state endemic diseases and the basic reproductive number, we can determine what interventions could help us shift the effective reproductive number below a critical value of 1. To illustrate how to use the Kermack-McKendrick model to assist us in designing disease interventions, we can take the classical example of a measles epidemic.

Suppose you're working for UNICEF's vaccine procurement division in a resource-poor area in which people have not been vaccinated against measles. A measles outbreak from a neighboring region has been reported. You want to know how many people in your area must be reached by your vaccination program to prevent an epidemic if an infected person crosses the border from the neighboring region into your area.

To prevent an epidemic, how many people in your area do you need to vaccinate before the infection arrives? Well, if R_0 is the number of susceptible people who will be infected by each infectious person in the fully susceptible population, then the effective reproductive number $R = R_0(1 - f)$ will be the number of susceptible people who will be infected in a population where fraction f of the population has been vaccinated before the infection arrived.

Hence, we need to make $R_0(1 - f) < 1$ to prevent an epidemic. Solving for f, we get Equation 9.23:

$$f > 1 - \frac{1}{R_0}.$$

[Equation 9.23]

For example, if we live in an area with 100,000 people and are trying to prevent a disease with $R_0 = 8.6$, then, to prevent an epidemic, the number of people who need to be vaccinated before an infected person comes from the neighboring region would be $1 - 1/8.6 = 0.88$, or 88%. We don't need to vaccinate 100% of people because of *herd immunity*, or the fact that susceptible people will be effectively surrounded by immune people if a sufficient number of people are vaccinated, thus preventing infected and susceptible people from being in sufficient contact to lead to propagation of an epidemic.

Suppose a person living in your area asks: "What's the chance that I will get infected if the disease comes here?" Well, suppose p is the probability that a person in the population becomes infected at some point (between now and time infinity, meaning some time far in the future). Then, using our hazard functions in Equation 9.5, the probability that the person is never infected (always escapes infection) is:

$$\lim_{t \to \infty} S(t) = e^{-\int_0^\infty \lambda(t)dt} = 1 - p.$$

[Equation 9.24]

Hence:

$$p = 1 - e^{-\int_0^\infty \lambda(t)dt} = 1 - e^{-\int_0^\infty \beta I(t)dt}.$$

[Equation 9.25]

The right-hand side of this equation can be further simplified. The integral of $I(t)$ from time 0 to time infinity is the total time spent infected by all people who were ever infected, which is the product of the people who were ever infectious ($N*p$, in a population of size N) and the time they spent being infected ($E(T_I) = 1/\nu$). So:

$$\int_0^\infty \beta I(t)dt = \frac{\beta N p}{\nu} = R_0 p.$$ [Equation 9.26]

Hence, we can simplify Equation 9.25 to:

$$p = 1 - e^{-\int_0^\infty \beta I(t)dt} = 1 - e^{-R_0 p}.$$ [Equation 9.27]

Equation 9.27 tell us that if we have historical information about a disease, such as how many people got a disease in a past epidemic, then we can estimate R_0 without even knowing any of the parameters like β or ν, because Equation 9.27 simplifies to:

$$R_0 = \frac{-\ln(1-p)}{p}.$$ [Equation 9.28]

For example, historical data from Hong Kong indicate that about 76% of people were ultimately infected in a prior epidemic of influenza. Based on this data, and not knowing anything else about the disease, we could estimate the R_0 of the influenza strain that hit Hong Kong as $-\ln(1 - 0.76)/0.76 = 1.9$.

Conversely, if we had an estimate of R_0, then we could find the larger root of Equation 9.28 and solve for p. A simple way to do this is in Excel is to type the value of R_0 into cell A1, then type a guess for p into cell A2 (a large value such as 1 would help, to get the larger root of the equation), type the equation "=1-EXP(-A1 *A2)" into cell A3, and type "=A3-A2" into cell A4. We want cell A4 to equal 0 so that we have both sides of Equation 9.27 equal to each other. We can then use the "Goal Seek" command under "Tools," in which we want to set the cell A4 to the value of 0 by changing the cell value of cell B2 (p).

Implementing the Kermack-McKendrick Model in Excel

To implement the Kermack-McKendrick model in Excel, we follow a similar procedure to the one we followed to implement Markov models in Excel.

First, we should recognize that Equations 9.15 through 9.17 can be converted from differential equations to *difference equations*, which simply interpret the number of people in a given state as the sum of the number of people in the state during a previous time step, plus the people entering during a given time step, minus the people exiting during the time step. The number entering or exiting during a time step will be the number affected by an entry/exit rate, multiplied by the entry/exit rate, multiplied by the time step Δt:

$$S(t+\Delta t)=S(t)+\mu N\Delta t-\beta I(t)S(t)\Delta t-\mu S(t)\Delta t \qquad \text{[Equation 9.29]}$$

$$I(t+\Delta t)=I(t)+\beta I(t)S(t)\Delta t-vI(t)\Delta t-\mu I(t)\Delta t \qquad \text{[Equation 9.30]}$$

$$R(t+\Delta t)=R(t)+vI(t)\Delta t-\mu R(t)\Delta t. \qquad \text{[Equation 9.31]}$$

Readers can download an Excel spreadsheet from this book's website (https://github.com/sanjaybasu/modelinghealthsystems), in which these equations have been implemented. As with our Markov models, we split the Kermack-McKendrick model simulation into two components: the input parameter table and the equations that simulate the number of people in a given state at any given time.

Suppose that our input parameters are a total population size of N = 100,000, with a birth/death rate if μ = 1/75 years^{-1}, a transmission probability per person of β = 0.000171, and a recovery rate of v = 2 years^{-1}.

In our example spreadsheet, we first typed these values into a table on the upper left, as shown in Figure 9.3.

Second, we need to create a time column. While our rate units are in years^{-1}, we are trying to simulate differential equations using difference equations and therefore should use very small time steps to simulate small values of Δt and thereby closely approximate the differential equations. We can choose 0.01 as a time step value, and

	A	B	C	D	E	F	G
1	N	100000		time	S	I	R
2	mu	0.01333333		0	99999	1	0
3	beta	0.000171		0.01	99998.82914	1.15086496	0.02
4	v	2		0.02	99998.6325	1.32448981	0.04301463
5	delta t	0.01		0.03	99998.40619	1.52430808	0.06949869
6				0.04	99998.14575	1.7542712	0.09997559
7				0.05	99997.84603	2.01892669	0.13504768
8				0.06	99997.50108	2.32350799	0.17540821
9				0.07	99997.10411	2.67403797	0.22185498
10				0.08	99996.64725	3.07744792	0.27530616
11				0.09	99996.12147	3.54171459	0.33681841

FIGURE 9.3 Implementation of the Kermack-McKendrick "SIR" model in Excel. The book website contains a version of the spreadsheet for download. As with our Markov models, we split the Kermack-McKendrick model simulation into two components: the input parameter table, and the equations that simulate the number of people in a given state at any given time.

therefore we also add Δt to our parameter table in cell B5. We have entered a column of times, as shown in Figure 9.3, in which the first time in cell D2 was time "0" and cell D3 was the formula "=D2+B$5"; we clicked and dragged cell D3 to produce a total of 5 years of simulation time. Note that we include dollar signs ($) around the 5 of B5 corresponding to Δt, ensuring that Excel always refers to the correct cell when we click and drag the formula down the time column.

Third, we set the initial conditions. We created three columns corresponding to our three states of disease: S, I, and R. In the initial time zero (row 2), we assume that everyone is susceptible except for just 1 person who is infected, such that we have 99,999 susceptible people, 1 infected person, and 0 recovered people.

Finally, we add in the difference equations. For the susceptible people in time point 0.01 (row 3), we read from Equation 9.29 and add the people who are susceptible in the prior time step (prior row) to the quantity $\mu N \Delta t - \beta I(t)S(t)\Delta(t) - \mu S(t)\Delta t$. In our Excel spreadsheet, this corresponds to typing in the expression "=E2+B$2*B$1*B$5-B$3*E2*F2*B$5-B$2*E2*B$5." Note again that we have included the dollars signs ($) around all expressions in our parameter table to ensure that Excel refers to the correct parameter when we click and drag the formula down all 5 simulated years. Also note that it is easy to forget the Δt (cell B5) in our formula, which is critical to ensure we accurately reflect the change in people among states over a small time interval.

For the infected people in time point 0.01 (row 3), we analogously read from Equation 9.30 and add the people who are infected in the prior time step (prior row) to the quantity $\beta I(t)S(t)\Delta(t) - \nu I(t)\Delta t - \mu I(t)\Delta t$, which corresponds to typing in the expression "=F2+B$3*E2*F2*B$5-B$4*F2*B$5-B$2*F2*B$5."

Finally, for the recovered people in time point 0.01 (row 3), we read from Equation 9.31 and add the people who are infected in the prior time step (prior row) to the quantity $\nu I(t)\Delta t - \mu R(t)\Delta t$, which corresponds to typing in the expression "=G2+B$4*F2*B$5-B$2*G2*B$5."

We can do a quick check to ensure our formulas produce a row of numbers adding to $N = 100,000$ people, meaning that we have not accidentally created or destroyed people in our constant population model.

When we click and drag our formulas for the S, I, and R states down through time point 10, Excel should simulate the overall epidemic. By highlighting the four columns from time through state R and inserting a scatterplot (click on the Insert menu, then Chart, then "X Y (Scatter)"), we obtain Figure 9.4.

We see from the figure that our model incorporating an infectious process produces a very complex result. First, we have a nonlinear increase in the number of infected people, which peaks and then slows down back to a final value of zero. Note that the population of infected people decreases naturally, without us doing

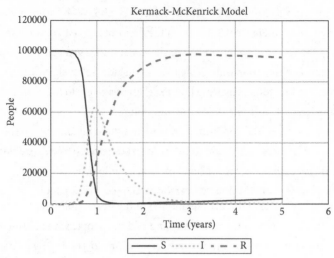

FIGURE 9.4 **Graph of the SIR model in Excel.**

anything; hence, we should not interpret the natural decline as an indication that our disease control efforts are successful. The susceptible population declines but then starts to increase gradually again as new people are born, being available in the future to spark another epidemic potentially. The recovered population similarly increases to include the whole population, but, as immune people die, the population in the recovered state diminishes.

Now that we have simulated a non–steady-state epidemic, we can answer several important questions about the disease. First, what is the highest prevalence of infected people that would be expected to occur during the epidemic? We can quickly identify the answer to this question by looking at the column of infected people and, in any cell, typing in the expression "=MAX(F:F)" where MAX is the Excel expression identifying the maximum value of the column F. In our simulation, the maximum prevalence equals 64,165 people. Scrolling through our column of infected people, we see this value corresponds to year 0.96, relatively early in the epidemic.

Conversely, what is the highest incidence of disease during any one time step? To find this value, we have to create a new column, with value $\beta I(t)S(t)dt$. If we type in this quantity, we see that the highest incidence is 3,599 cases per time step and occurs in year 0.8. The maximum prevalence time step doesn't correspond to the maximum incident time step since it takes time for incidence to manifest as a higher prevalence (i.e., several days of high incidence will build up into high incidence before the prevalence subsequently declines through recovery).

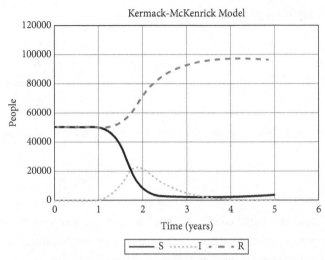

FIGURE 9.5 **Graph of the SIR model in Excel, after introducing a vaccination program.**

Now we can model a vaccination program and examine how that might affect our epidemic. Suppose we vaccinate some fraction of people before the epidemic starts. We can add a new parameter to our table, parameter f, and set it to an arbitrary initial value of 50% (in cell B6 for our example spreadsheet). We can then modify our model to incorporate the fraction vaccinated by modifying the equation for susceptible and recovered people. Namely, fraction $(1 - f)$ of people who were previously susceptible will enter the susceptible state, while fraction f of people who were previously susceptible will enter the recovered state. Hence, we can replace our initial condition for state S with the equation "=99,999*(1-B6)" and state R with the equation "=99,999*B6."

We can then adjust the value of the fraction f to examine how increased vaccination levels before the epidemic began would alter the overall shape of the epidemic curve. Figure 9.5 shows the overall epidemic shape when the vaccinated fraction is 50%.

IMPLEMENTING THE KERMACK-MCKENDRICK MODEL IN *R*

An example of *R* code to program the model is provided on this book's website (https://github.com/sanjaybasu/modelinghealthsystems). To program the Kermack-McKendrick model in *R*, we specify the same key elements that we specified for the Excel model: the parameters that will go into our equations, how long we want to run the simulation, the initial conditions, and the equations themselves.

First, we input our parameters:

```
N = 100000
mu = 1/75
beta = 0.000171
v = 2
```

Second, we specify how long we want to run the model and with what time steps:

```
time = 5
dt = 0.01
```

Third, we input our initial conditions. We'll also create some vectors named after each state, which we'll later expand for future time points, but which for now will only contain the initial conditions:

```
S = 99999
I = 1
R = 0

Svec = S
Ivec = I
Rvec = R
```

Finally, we write our equations and insert them into two "for loops" to have R update over each period of time (first for loop) and across all small time steps (second for loop). In each loop, we concatenate (add on) the current value of the state to the list of previous values, expanding the vector with each time step across all simulated time points. Note that there are more efficient ways to code this using the library "deSolve," but this way is more intuitive for learning purposes:

```
for (i in 1:time){
  for (i in 1:(1/dt)){
    S = S + mu*N*dt - beta*S*I*dt - mu*S*dt
    I = I + beta*S*I*dt - v*I*dt - mu*I*dt
    R = R + v*I*dt - mu*R*dt
    Svec = c(Svec, S)
    Ivec = c(Ivec, I)
    Rvec = c(Rvec, R)
  }
}
```

Now we can plot the result; here, we use the Quick-R website (http://www.stat-methods.net/graphs/line.html) to remind ourselves of how to color the lines blue (col="blue"), choose a smooth line (type="l"), and label our axes (xlab="time steps", ylab="Pop"). We choose one vector to start the plot with the plot command, then add the other two lines using the lines command:

```
plot(Svec,col="blue",type="l",xlab="time steps",ylab="Pop")
lines(Ivec,col="red")
lines(Rvec,col="green")
```

The Quick-R site also reminds us how to add a legend by specifying the x-axis location for the left corner of the legend box, the y-axis location for the top of the legend box, the labels for the legend, the type of lines we want in the legend, and the colors.:

```
legend(400,80000,c("S","I","R"),lty=c(1,1,1),col=c("blue",
"red","green"))
```

The plot commands produce Figure 9.6.

We can use the power of R to extend the model to do something we simply don't have the ability to do in Excel: create a large-scale uncertainty analysis. Suppose that we don't know exactly what the value of the input parameters are. We might know, for example, that $\beta = 0.000171$ on average but with a standard deviation of 0.00001, and $v = 2$ on average but with a standard deviation of 0.1.

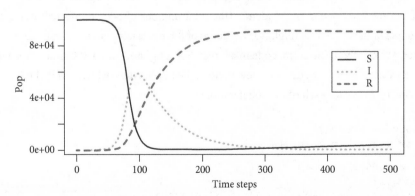

FIGURE 9.6 **Graph of the SIR model in R. The book website contains a version of the code for download.**

How much would this affect the number of people infected in the first year of the epidemic?

We can first create a vector to keep track of how many total people get infected over the 1-year simulation by adding a vector *Totinf* = *0* before the "for loop" and adding within the for loop the code:

```
Totvec = c(Totvec, beta*S*I*dt)
```

This code keeps track of how many people are newly infected in each time step. Hence, the sum from time 0 to time 1/dt will be the total number of people infected over the course of the first year of the epidemic:

```
> sum(Totvec)
[1] 101842.4
```

Next, we can make our model *stochastic* instead of *deterministic*. That is, rather than having the value of the parameters predetermined at set values, we can have the model incorporate parameters that are stochastic, or chosen from random distributions we specify. In this case, our initial parameters will now be:

```
N = 100000
mu = 1/75
beta = rnorm(1,mean=0.000171,sd=0.00003)
v = rnorm(1,mean=2,sd=0.2)
```

The rnorm commands indicate that *R* should sample once from a normal distribution with means and standard deviations as specified. Now, we want to know how much the final size of the epidemic (the total number of people infected over the course of the epidemic) might vary because of the uncertainty in the parameter values. We can wrap the entire code in a larger "for loop" and run it 100 times, storing the value of sum(Totvec) in a new vector called *Totveciters*, which will include the value of *Totvec* for each of the 100 iterations:

```
Totveciters=c()
for (iters in 1:100){

N = 100000
mu = 1/75
beta = rnorm(1,mean=0.000171,sd=0.00001)
v = rnorm(1,mean=2,sd=0.1)

time = 1
dt = 0.01
```

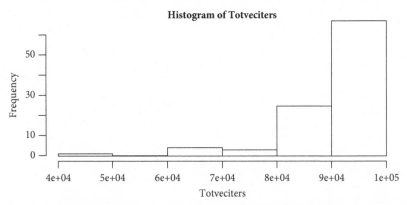

FIGURE 9.7 The histogram that tells us how much the size of our epidemic in the first year varied due to the uncertainty in our input parameters. The x-axis displays the value of 'Totveciters', or the total number of people infected over the course of the first year of the simulated epidemic across multiple simulated iterations of the model. The y-axis displays the frequency of each value of Totveciters.

```
S = 99999
I = 1
R = 0

Svec = S
Ivec = I
Rvec = R
Totvec = 0

for (i in 1:time){
  for (i in 1:(1/dt)){
    S = S + mu*N*dt - beta*S*I*dt - mu*S*dt
    I = I + beta*S*I*dt - v*I*dt - mu*I*dt
    R = R + v*I*dt - mu*R*dt
    Svec = c(Svec, S)
      Rvec = c(Rvec, R)
    Totvec = c(Totvec, beta*S*I*dt)
  }
}
plot(Svec,col="blue",type="l",xlab="time steps",ylab="Pop")
lines(Ivec,col="red")
lines(Rvec,col="green")
legend(400,80000,c("S","I","R"),lty=c(1,1,1),col=c("blue","re
d","green"))

Totveciters=c(Totveciters,sum(Totvec))
}
```

We can finally plot the histogram that tells us how much the size of our epidemic in the first year varied due to the uncertainty in our input parameters, which is shown in Figure 9.7.

10

COMPLEXITIES OF EPIDEMIC MODELING

In the prior chapter, we derived and simulated the most basic epidemic model. We assumed that people can be in only one of three states (susceptible, infected, or recovered) and that people mix homogeneously throughout the population. In this chapter, we examine how the Kermack-McKendrick model can be extended to simulate a wide variety of complex diseases and circumstances and be adapted to incorporate the complex ways that people contact each other. We additionally describe methods for simulating individual behavior in response to an epidemic.

EXTENDING THE STANDARD KERMACK-MCKENDRICK MODEL

Once we leave the context of the Kermack-McKendrick model, the calculation of R_0 unfortunately becomes complicated—often too complicated to produce any simple formulas that are memorable enough to be recalled for day-to-day public health practice. (Note that the R_0 can still be calculated using mathematics that are beyond the level of this work, as detailed elsewhere.[1]) Because of this, we often have to resort to simulation to identify what effect a disease will have in a population and to measure the potential impact of a public health intervention on the disease.

We can extend our basic Kermack-McKendrick model simulation to incorporate a wide variety of diseases and interventions. Suppose, for example, that we want to model two potential interventions to reduce the burden of tuberculosis (TB). People who are infected with TB are not always infectious. Rather, people go into a "dormant" or "latent" state of disease (which is not dangerous and not infectious), sometimes for several decades, before "activating" to the form of active lung disease that we commonly associate with TB (and which is both infectious and potentially fatal if untreated).

As a public health planner, you want to compare two different strategies for reducing the burden of TB: (1) investment in a program to find and treat people with latent TB, thus preventing them from transitioning to active TB sometime in the future; and (2) investment in a program to expand treatment for people with active TB, thus preventing them from infecting susceptible people.

There is no way to compare these programs using the standard Kermack-McKendrick model, but we can extend the model to address the unique pathogenesis of TB. We can approach the problem with the same strategy we have used for all of our models: first draw the model diagram, then write down equations describing the diagram.

Our model diagram is shown in Figure 10.1. In the diagram, we have extended the classical Kermack-McKendrick model to account for the unique nature of TB. Here, we have extended the Kermack-McKendrick model to a "SEIR model," which extends the SIR structure by adding a group of "exposed" people between the susceptible and infectious group. The exposed group is latently infected, but not yet infectious. They can move on to the infectious state at some rate γ. Also, since TB is a potentially deadly disease, suppose that there is a rate of death κ from the active, infectious state.

We can write down a series of equations based on our model diagram:

$$\frac{dS(t)}{dt} = \mu N(t) - \beta I(t) S(t) - \mu S(t) \qquad \text{[Equation 10.1]}$$

$$\frac{dE(t)}{dt} = \beta I(t) S(t) - \gamma E(t) - \mu E(t) \qquad \text{[Equation 10.2]}$$

$$\frac{dI(t)}{dt} = \gamma E(t) - v I(t) - \kappa I(t) - \mu I(t) \qquad \text{[Equation 10.3]}$$

$$\frac{dR(t)}{dt} = v I(t) - \mu R(t). \qquad \text{[Equation 10.4]}$$

There are several differences between the SEIR model and the Kermack-McKendrick SIR model. First, we see that we have added one equation for the exposed (latent) TB

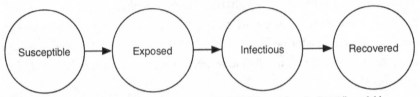

FIGURE 10.1 Expection of the Kermack-McKendrick "SIR" model to the "SEIR" model by addition of the "exposed" state, which is not infectious but can progress to an infectious state.

state. People enter that state from the susceptible class and flow to the active TB state at the rate γ. We have additionally added a rate of death from TB of κ from the active, infectious state. Hence, we should not expect to have a constant population size in our model.

This book's website has the R code corresponding to this model (https://github.com/sanjaybasu/modelinghealthsystems). Because the course of TB epidemics takes a long time to simulate, it would be painful to simulate in Excel (requiring hundreds of rows of equations); hence, we will implement the code in R for ease. The code utilizes the following set of parameters: $N = 100,000$ people, $\beta = 0.001$, $\mu = 1/75$ years^{-1}, $\gamma = 0.05$ years^{-1}, $v = 2$ years^{-1}, and $\kappa = 0.1$ years^{-1} (note that we are using convenient round numbers here and elsewhere in the book for teaching purposes; these parameters should not be misconstrued to reflect actual TB epidemics). We also set the initial conditions such that S = 99,999 people, E = 0 people, I = 1 person, and R = 0 people.

As in Chapter 9, we begin our R model code by first specifying our parameters:

```
N = 100000
beta = 0.001
mu = 1/75
gamma = 0.05
v = 2
kappa = 0.1
```

Second, we declare our time horizon of interest, let's say 20 years, and a small time step:

```
time = 20
dt = 0.01
```

Third, we insert our initial conditions and initiate some vectors for each state:

```
S = 99999
E = 0
I = 1
R = 0

Svec = S
Evec = E
Ivec = I
Rvec = R
```

Fourth, we insert our equations in two "for loops" (the first spanning across all times and the second loop for each small time step within each time period). The current state in each loop is then added to the vectors for each state:

```
for (i in 1:time){
  for (i in 1:(1/dt)){
    S = S + mu*N*dt - beta*S*I*dt - mu*S*dt
    E = E + beta*S*I*dt - gamma*E*dt - mu*E*dt
    I = I + gamma*E*dt - v*I*dt - kappa*I*dt - mu*I*dt
    R = R + v*I*dt - mu*R*dt
    Svec = c(Svec, S)
    Evec = c(Evec, E)
    Ivec = c(Ivec, I)
    Rvec = c(Rvec, R)
    N = S+E+I+R
  }
}
```

Note that we have updated the total population size *N* with each time step since we are no longer assuming a constant population size because TB is deadly.

Finally, we can plot our results, adding the exposed group to our plot in purple, as shown in Figure 10.2.

```
plot(Svec,col="blue",type="l",xlab="time  steps",ylab="Pop",yl
im=c(0,100000))
lines(Evec,col="purple")
lines(Ivec,col="red")
lines(Rvec,col="green")
legend(1500,100000,c("S","E","I","R"),lty=c(1,1,1,1),col=c("b
lue","purple","red","green"))
```

As with our Kermack-McKendrick model in Chapter 9, we first plot one vector, specifying its color, line type, labels, and limits of the y-axis (from 0 to 100,000 people in this case). Then we plot other vectors as lines and add a legend, specifying the legend's position, text, line types, and colors; the commands produce Figure 10.2.

We see in Figure 10.2 that the curves for the disease are very different from the original Kermack-McKendrick model. The disease spreads over a longer period of time. Many people become latently infected, although only a few are actively infectious. Because Figure 10.2 is zoomed out, we can't see the infected line very clearly. Hence, we can just plot the infectious group by themselves:

```
plot(Ivec,col="red",type="l",xlab="time steps",ylab="Pop")
```

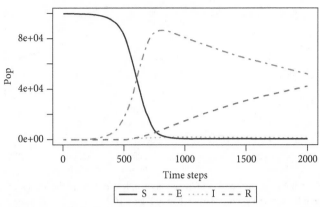

FIGURE 10.2 Simulation of the SEIR model in R. Curves for the disease are very different from the original Kermack-McKendrick model. The x-axis reflects time steps (1/100 of the year) in the simulation, and the y-axis reflects the number of people in the model in each state. The variables "S", "E", "I", and "R" reflect each of the four states of disease shown in Figure 10.1.

This produces Figure 10.3, where we see an interesting shape to the infectious pool, which peaks at a prevalence of about 2,000 people, with a very gradual rise and an even slower fall:

```
> max(Ivec)
[1] 2019.316
```

We can compare the two interventions we hope to contrast: (1) investment in a program to find and treat people with latent TB, thus preventing them from transitioning to active TB sometime in the future; and (2) investment in a program to expand treatment for people with active TB, thus preventing them from infecting susceptible people. Let's suppose that investment in treating people with latent TB would add a new rate that would remove people from the exposed state and put them in the recovered state at a rate $\tau = 0.1$ year^{-1}. Let's say that, by contrast, more investment in expanding treatment would increase the recovery rate to a value of 5 year^{-1}. Which program would make more impact on the total number of people who die from tuberculosis over the next 20 years?

For the treatment of latent TB, we can modify the equations slightly to add on the rate $\tau = 0.1$ year^{-1} shifting people from the latent to the recovered state. We first add the code:

```
tau = 0.1
```

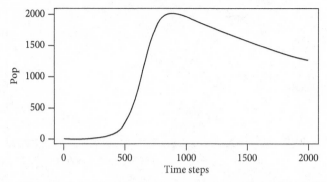

FIGURE 10.3 **Change in the number of infectious people over time in the SEIR model implemented in R. Note the y-axis is larger than in Figure 10.2.**

We can include the code defining tau with the other parameters at the beginning of the code. We can then modify the equations to reflect the new rate of flow from the exposed to the recovered state:

```
S = S + mu*N*dt - beta*S*I*dt - mu*S*dt
E = E + beta*S*I*dt - gamma*E*dt - mu*E*dt - tau*E*dt
I = I + gamma*E*dt - v*I*dt - kappa*I*dt - mu*I*dt
R = R + v*I*dt - mu*R*dt + tau*E*dt
```

We next need to determine what the overall number of people who die from TB would be over the time period, which is 20 years. We can add one more vector before the "for loop" to hold this quantity:

```
Deaths = 0
```

Then we can update its value within the "for loop":

```
Deaths = c(Deaths, kappa*I*dt)
```

When we run the model, we see that the total deaths after introducing the latent TB treatment program is about 1,400:

```
> sum(Deaths)
[1] 1398.232
```

Next, we can compare the number of deaths to the situation if we increased the recovery rate to a value of 3 year^{-1}. We first set the value of τ to 0, to show the absence of the latent treatment case, then set the value of v to 5. Running the model in this scenario, we see that the total number of deaths has been dramatically reduced, to just under 700:

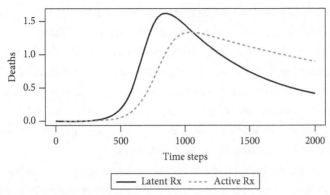

FIGURE 10.4 **Change to the numbers of deaths from tuberculosis based on the SEIR model, if we treat latently-infected persons or if we treat active infectious people.**

```
> sum(Deaths)
[1] 681.6078
```

The comparison between the two treatment alternatives can be visualized in Figure 10.4.

Our example reveals that we can extend the Kermack-McKendrick model in several ways to accommodate a variety of diseases and interventions. In addition to adding new states, we can add new flows between states. We can quickly extend the model in *R* and define the metrics we want to compare. In the next section, we'll also look at how to relax a key assumption we've used so far: The Law of Mass Action, which assumed that people are homogeneously mixing together and thereby all share roughly the same risk.

HETEROGENEOUS MIXING

Up to this point, we've been assuming *homogeneous mixing* of a population—meaning that people contact one another at a relatively even rate throughout the population, such that every person experiences the same average rate of disease. That's often a pretty good approximation to understand the general trends in large populations, but in some cases—for example, in the case of many sexually transmitted diseases (STDs)—we need to modify that assumption. In the case of STDs, some people who have minimal amounts of sexual contact will be at very low risk for disease, while others who change sexual partners frequently will be at much higher risk. Many other diseases that present a major public health burden also involve such *heterogeneous mixing*, such as diseases that travel via injection drug use or diseases that are segregated to only the poorest or most crowded areas of cities. Public health workers take a great deal of care to find the target population for their interventions, which often means determining those people who are at highest risk for disease and providing both preventative and therapeutic interventions to them.

It has been observed that the American population tends to cluster around sexual activity "classes," in which a majority of people had a low level of sexual activity and a smaller pool of people have very high rates of activity. A question has been whether it is more worthwhile to focus many resources on a few people at the high end of the activity distribution or whether a more even spread of resources across more people would result in broader benefits at the population-level.

To address the dilemma of whether targeting treatment or broadening treatment might have more impact, let's build a model to simulate a simple heterosexually transmitted STD. Suppose we want a model of a disease like gonorrhea, in which infected/infectious people can be treated and return to the susceptible state, meaning that, instead of an SIR model, we just have an SI model.

As with any other model, we can start the modeling process by drawing a diagram describing our model, followed by a set of equations translating our diagram into symbols.

In Figure 10.5, we have drawn an SI model but created four subsets of persons for each of the four subsets of a heterosexual STD epidemic: high-activity men, high-activity women, low-activity men, and low-activity women. We end up with eight states to draw because we have two states of disease for each of two sexes, for each of two classes of sexual activity.

Since we are only simulating heterosexual transmission of the STD, we will have the rate of infection among men depend on the prevalence of infected women, and the rate of infection among women depend on the prevalence of infected men.

But a key challenge is how we can model the transmission rate. We need some strategy to overcome the Law of Mass Action. Rather than simply providing an estimate of the transmission risk coefficient β for all people, we need to account for the differences in risk levels between the high-activity and low-activity classes.

One strategy to account for the complex mixing of people would be to break up the general transmission risk coefficient β into three component parts: (1) a part that has to do with the rate of risky contact (e.g., unprotected sexual encounters per year); (2) a second part that has to do with the biology of the organism being analyzed (e.g., the probability of transmission of the organism from one person to another, per unprotected sexual encounter between a susceptible and an infected person); and (3) a third part, which captures the probability of mixing with a person of the same or different activity level (e.g., is transmission from a high-activity or low-activity person). Let's say that the rate of unprotected contact is variable c, the

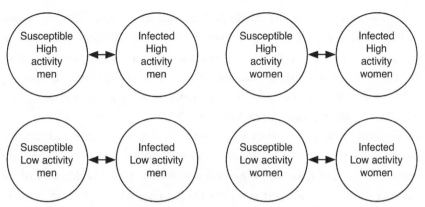

FIGURE 10.5 The susceptible-infected model of a heterosexually-sexually-transmitted disease.

probability of transmission of the organism from an infected to a susceptible person per unprotected contact is p, and the probability of mixing with a person of the same or different class is w. Hence, $\beta = c^*p^*w$. An advantage of breaking up one variable into two components, in this case, is that the interventions that we'll model may alter the rate of risky contact (e.g., educational interventions) and/or the probability of transmission (e.g., condom use), hence the extra complexity is justified since we know what the impact of STD-related interventions are on these parameters, but we don't know their effect on a generic transmission rate β.

Furthermore, it's not simply the case that highly active people interact with people who have high activity, and vice versa. Otherwise, we would have two different populations of people altogether; to the contrary, there are a proportion of people who mix between the two groups. This can be represented by a matrix, often called the "contact matrix," "mixing matrix," or "who acquires infection from whom" (WAIFW) matrix. Table 10.1 provides an example of a WAIFW matrix, which we note is not symmetrical because, from the perspective of a high-activity person, the chances of encountering another highly active person is much greater than the probability of encountering a low-activity person.

To refer to this matrix, we can use conventional notation w[row, column], such that w[1,1] means the probability that a low-activity person has unprotected sex

Table 10.1 Example of a who acquires infection from whom (WAIFW) matrix

Contact Matrix (w)	Probability Each Sexual Encounter Is with:	
Subject:	Low-Activity Person	High-Activity Person
Low-Activity Person	0.6	0.4
High-Activity Person	0.1	0.9

with a low-activity person, 0.6. Similarly, w[1,2] means the probability that a low-activity person has sex with a high-activity person, 0.4. If the matrix were different between men and women, we could use two matrices (one for each gender), but we can assume the same matrix for men and women for simplicity in this example.

Next, we write down equations for our model. Looking at our model diagram, we will have eight equations for each of the eight categories of people, where we can use the subscript m to refer to men, f to refer to women, h to refer to high-activity, and j to refer to low-activity. For simplicity, we will also assume that birth and death are such small rates from the perspective of a short-term STD epidemic that we will omit those rates from these equations and just focus on infection and recovery (rate v):

$$\frac{dS_{m,h}}{dt} = -pc_h\left(w[2,1]I_{f,j} + w[2,2]I_{f,h}\right) + vI_{m,h} \qquad \text{[Equation 10.5]}$$

$$\frac{dI_{m,h}}{dt} = +pc_h\left(w[2,1]I_{f,j} + w[2,2]I_{f,h}\right) - vI_{m,h} \qquad \text{[Equation 10.6]}$$

$$\frac{dS_{f,h}}{dt} = -pc_h\left(w[2,1]I_{m,j} + w[2,2]I_{m,h}\right) + vI_{f,h} \qquad \text{[Equation 10.7]}$$

$$\frac{dI_{f,h}}{dt} = +pc_h\left(w[2,1]I_{m,j} + w[2,2]I_{m,h}\right) - vI_{f,h} \qquad \text{[Equation 10.8]}$$

$$\frac{dS_{m,j}}{dt} = -pc_j\left(w[1,1]I_{f,j} + w[1,2]I_{f,h}\right) + vI_{m,j} \qquad \text{[Equation 10.9]}$$

$$\frac{dI_{m,j}}{dt} = +pc_j\left(w[1,1]I_{f,j} + w[1,2]I_{f,h}\right) - vI_{m,j} \qquad \text{[Equation 10.10]}$$

$$\frac{dS_{f,j}}{dt} = -pc_j\left(w[1,1]I_{m,j} + w[1,2]I_{m,h}\right) + vI_{f,j} \qquad \text{[Equation 10.11]}$$

$$\frac{dI_{f,j}}{dt} = +pc_j\left(w[1,1]I_{m,j} + w[1,2]I_{m,h}\right) - vI_{f,j}. \qquad \text{[Equation 10.12]}$$

In each equation, we see that the infection rate is a product of the biological probability of transmission upon an unprotected encounter, the rate of such encounters (conditional on the activity class of the person), the probability that the infected person being contacted is of one class or another, and the prevalence of infection among such persons. This book's website has accompanying R code to implement this model (https://github.com/sanjaybasu/modelinghealthsystems). As with prior models, we begin the model with the input parameters, which in this case include a contact vector with two components (a value of 5 per year for high-risk people and 1 per year for low-risk people), and a WAIFW matrix:

```
p = 0.44
c = c(5,1)
w = matrix(c(.6,.4,.1,.9),ncol=2,byrow=TRUE)
v=2
```

We next set the time horizon for the model and the time steps:

```
time = 10
dt = 0.01
```

As with other models, we specify initial conditions and starting vectors for our states; in this case, we have arbitrarily split the population into 50% males and 50% females, with 10% of each sex in the high-activity class:

```
Smh = 4999
Imh = 1
Sfh = 4999
Ifh = 1
Smj = 44999
Imj = 1
Sfj = 44999
Ifj = 1

Smhvec = Smh
Imhvec = Imh
Sfhvec = Sfh
Ifhvec = Ifh
Smjvec = Smj
Imjvec = Imj
Sfjvec = Sfj
Ifjvec = Ifj
```

Inside our "for loop," we insert the equations just as they appear in Equations 10.5 through 10.12, but using R's ability to look up the c vector and w matrix to find the right parameters for each group of people:

```
for (i in 1:time){
  for (i in 1:(1/dt)){

    Smh = Smh-p*c[1]*(w[2,1]*Ifj+w[2,2]*Ifh)*dt+v*Imh*dt
    Imh = Imh+p*c[1]*(w[2,1]*Ifj+w[2,2]*Ifh)*dt-v*Imh*dt
```

```
Sfh = Sfh-p*c[1]*(w[2,1]*Imj+w[2,2]*Imh)*dt+v*Ifh*dt
Ifh = Ifh+p*c[1]*(w[2,1]*Imj+w[2,2]*Imh)*dt-v*Ifh*dt
Smj = Smj-p*c[2]*(w[1,1]*Ifj+w[1,2]*Ifh)*dt+v*Imj*dt
Imj = Imj+p*c[2]*(w[1,1]*Ifj+w[1,2]*Ifh)*dt-v*Imj*dt
Sfj = Sfj-p*c[2]*(w[1,1]*Imj+w[1,2]*Imh)*dt+v*Ifj*dt
Ifj = Ifj+p*c[2]*(w[1,1]*Imj+w[1,2]*Imh)*dt-v*Ifj*dt
Smhvec = c(Smhvec,Smh)
Imhvec = c(Imhvec,Imh)
Sfhvec = c(Sfhvec,Sfh)
Ifhvec = c(Ifhvec,Ifh)
Smjvec = c(Smjvec,Smj)
Imjvec = c(Imjvec,Imj)
Sfjvec = c(Sfjvec,Sfj)
Ifjvec = c(Ifjvec,Ifj)
  }
}
```

Finally, after our "for loop," we can plot the fraction of each group that becomes infected over each time step:

```
plot(Imhvec/(Smhvec+Imhvec),col="blue",type="l",xlab="time
steps",ylab="Pop",ylim=c(0,1))
lines(Ifhvec/(Sfhvec+Ifhvec),col="purple")
lines(Imjvec/(Smjvec+Imjvec),col="red")
lines(Ifjvec/(Sfjvec+Ifjvec),col="green")
legend(800,1,c("MH","FH","MJ","FJ"),lty=c(1,1,1,1),col=c("blue",
"purple","red","green"))
```

As shown in Figure 10.6, the high-activity group reaches a steady-state fraction of infection with about 23.8% of them infected, while the low-activity group reaches a steady-state with only about 0.3% infected.

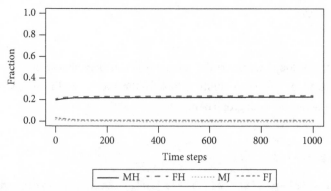

FIGURE 10.6 Fraction of people infected among "male, high-risk" (MH), "female high-risk" (FH), "male low-risk" (MJ) and "female low-risk" (FJ) people in the susceptible-infected model of a heterosexually-sexually-transmitted disease. Note that the lines for MH and FH overlap, as do the lines for MJ and FJ. The book website contains code in R to reproduce the graph.

Now that we developed a model to investigate the dynamics of the epidemic, we can compare various interventions to control the epidemic. Suppose we have two options as public health practitioners: we can either direct our program resources to target the high-activity subpopulation, or we can distribute the same resources broadly across the population. Based on empirical research studies, we estimate that if we target the high-activity subpopulation, we would decrease their rate of risky sex by about 20% (i.e., their parameter c lowers from 5 to 5*0.8 = 4). On the other hand, if we spread out our resources throughout the population, we'd have fewer resources to go around, so we'd decrease the rates of risky sex among both low-activity and high-activity groups by about 4% (i.e., the overall vector c = c(5,1)*0.96 = c(4.8, 0.96)). Which strategy should we pursue if we want to minimize total number of people infected in the population over the 10-year time horizon?

First, we can create a vector to track the number of people infected in the population over the 10-year time horizon. We can create an empty vector before the "for loop":

```
Numinf = 0
```

We can then insert an updating mechanism inside the "for loop":

```
Numinf = c(Numinf, p*c[1]*(w[2,1]*Ifj+w[2,2]*Ifh)*dt+p*c[1]*(w
[2,1]*Imj+w[2,2]*Imh)*dt+p*c[2]*(w[1,1]*Ifj+w[1,2]*Ifh)*dt+p*
c[2]*(w[1,1]*Imj+w[1,2]*Imh)*dt)
```

Finally, we can sum after the "for loop" to find our total number infected:

```
> sum(Numinf)
[1] 49872.04
```

Now that we have an estimate of the total infections, we can evaluate how our two interventions alter this total infection number. For the first intervention, we can reduce the parameter c corresponding only to the high-activity class from a value of 5 to a value of 4. Running the model under these conditions, we get a result of:

```
> sum(Numinf)
[1] 10178.38
```

For the second intervention, we can change the vector c to a value of c(4.8, 0.96), which produces:

```
> sum(Numinf)
[1] 32825.39
```

Hence, focusing on just the high-risk subpopulation would be expected to be massively more impactful than focusing a little bit on everyone, with less than one-third of infections produced over the course of 10 years.

Overall, the example of the STD epidemic shows us how a SIR model can be extended when we wish to depart from the Law of Mass Action and instead take into account a heterogeneous mixing matrix. As illustrated in this example, even a simple deviation to two classes of risk produces a large number of equations and complexities for modeling. An even more complex strategy for modeling heterogeneous transmission is the approach of simulating dynamic social networks and how they influence disease transmission. Although the mathematics of network simulation are beyond the scope of this book, the "EpiModel" package in R provides a user-friendly approach to simulate epidemics over networks and can be installed and utilized just like any other package to produce simulations of epidemics incorporating dynamic social networks.

VECTOR-BORNE DISEASE

Particularly in the context of climate change and rising temperatures that spread mosquitoes and other insects, infectious disease epidemiologists are increasingly concerned about the potential threat of increasing vector-borne (e.g., mosquito-driven) epidemics. When more than one species is involved in the spread of disease, it may not be obvious how we can adapt the Kermack-McKendrick model to address epidemics of vector-borne disease. Here, we illustrate how SIR-type models can be extended to address diseases where more than just the human species is involved.

Suppose, for example, that we wish to simulate the prevalence of malaria. We can simulate malaria as an SI model in which both humans and mosquitoes can be infected, as shown in Figure 10.7. Note that while humans can recover from infection, mosquitoes typically do not.

We can designate humans with subscript h and mosquitoes as subscript m. Humans catch malaria from mosquitoes, and mosquitoes catch malaria from humans. Translating these dynamics into equations, we have Equations 10.13 through 10.16:

$$\frac{dS_h}{dt} = \mu_h N_h + \nu I_h - \beta I_m S_h - \mu_h S_h \qquad \text{[Equation 10.13]}$$

$$\frac{dI_h}{dt} = \beta I_m S_h - \nu I_h - \kappa_h I_h - \mu_h I_h \qquad \text{[Equation 10.14]}$$

$$\frac{dS_m}{dt} = \mu_m N_m - \beta I_h S_m - \mu_m S_m \qquad \text{[Equation 10.15]}$$

$$\frac{dI_m}{dt} = \beta I_h S_m - \kappa_m I_m - \mu_m I_m. \qquad \text{[Equation 10.16]}$$

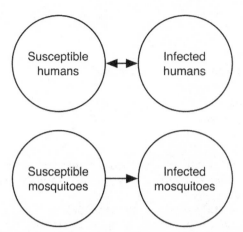

FIGURE 10.7 **Simulation of a malaria epidemic with susceptible and infectious humans and mosquitoes. While humans can recover from infection, mosquitoes typically do not.**

We can see that the first two equations describe an SI model among humans with recovery rate v and death rate from malaria κ. The rate of infection depends on the number of infected mosquitoes. Similarly, mosquitoes face an infection rate dependent on the number of infected humans. The R code corresponding to this model can be downloaded from this book's website. First, we used the following parameters vectors, where the first element of each vector is the parameter corresponding to humans, and the second is the parameter corresponding to mosquitoes, with time units in years:

```
mu = c(.015,12)
beta = 0.0003
kappa = c(1/5, 10)
v = 2
```

Second, we specify our time horizon and time step:

```
time = 1
dt = 0.0001
```

Here, we've intentionally chosen to simulate just 1 year in very small time steps to illustrate the complex dynamics between humans and mosquitoes.

Next, we specify our initial conditions and populate empty vectors:

```
Sh = 90000
Ih = 10000
Sm = 900000
Im = 100000

Shvec = Sh
Ihvec = Ih
```

```
Smvec = Sm
Imvec = Im
```

Finally, we insert our equations into a "for loop":

```
for (i in 1:time){
  for (i in 1:(1/dt)){
    Nh = Sh+Ih
    Nm = Sm+Im
    Sh = Sh + mu[1]*Nh*dt + v*Ih*dt - beta*Im*Sh*dt - mu[1]*Sh*dt
    Ih = Ih + beta*Im*Sh*dt - v*Ih*dt- kappa[1]*Ih*dt -
    mu[1]*Ih*dt
    Sm = Sm + mu[2]*Nm*dt - beta*Ih*Sm*dt - mu[2]*Sm*dt
    Im = Im + beta*Ih*Sm*dt - kappa[2]*Im*dt - mu[2]*Im*dt
    Shvec = c(Shvec,Sh)
    Ihvec = c(Ihvec,Ih)
    Smvec = c(Smvec,Sm)
    Imvec = c(Imvec,Im)
  }
}
```

When we insert commands to plot our output, we obtain Figure 10.8:

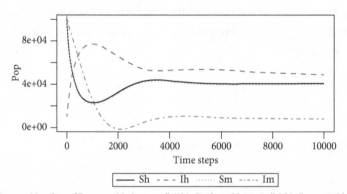

FIGURE 10.8 Number of "susceptible humans" (Sh), "infected humans" (Ih), "susceptible mosquitoes" (Sm) and "infected mosquitoes" (Im) in a simulated malaria epidemic. The book website contains code in *R* to reproduce the graph.

```
plot(Shvec,col="blue",type="l",xlab="time  steps",ylab="Pop",y
lim=c(0,500000))
lines(Ihvec,col="purple")
lines(Smvec,col="red")
lines(Imvec,col="green")
legend(7000,100000,c("Sh","Ih","Sm","Im"),lty=c(1,1,1,1),col=
c("blue","purple","red","green"))
```

We see that because humans and mosquitoes live on such different time scales, the prevalence of malaria tends to change wildly as the two species infect each other. One can further introduce seasonality by adjusting the birth rate of mosquitoes to be a sine function over time, enabling us to reintroduce more susceptible mosquitoes over time, in turn producing new waves of infection and a harmonic back-and-forth of infectious seasons.

Overall, we can see from this chapter that the Kermack-McKendrick model is not limited in its capacity but instead is quite versatile in how it can be extended to a wide range of infectious diseases and interventions, producing a complex and meaningful tool for public health planners to understand the complex dynamics of infectious diseases.

11

GOOD MODELING PRACTICES

Throughout this book, we have focused on the practices of constructing our own models or using standard modeling templates and strategies to solve common public health and healthcare system problems. But inherent to the task of using models is the challenge of being a good consumer of models. Often, we are faced with the task of reading and interpreting models produced by others and determining whether we "believe" the model results and can make use of the model implementation to help us make decisions. In this chapter, we address the issue of how we might become better consumers of modeling studies.

WHY MODELS ARE USEFUL, DESPITE
MAKING ASSUMPTIONS

Models are valuable for planning interventions that cannot be tested through randomized controlled trials (ethically or practically), simulating the implications of alternative theories about disease pathogenesis or control strategies, and estimating population-wide costs and consequences of public health programs. Since every public health policy decision implicitly involves assumptions, simply avoiding models because they present assumptions is not a logical approach to health policy. For example, even a "simple" policy to vaccinate children against an infectious disease makes several implicit assumptions: that the vaccine supply will be sufficient to generate herd immunity in the inoculated population, that the human and physical resources needed to administer the vaccine to the needy population are available and affordable, and that these resources are distributed in the population in a manner that maximizes benefits while minimizing costs. Modeling forces us to make these assumptions explicit and to compare how outcomes of interest might change if these assumptions were altered (e.g., How much more might it cost to reach populations that are currently far from health clinics?). Hence, models are highly useful precisely because they make explicit the dilemmas inherent to the public health policy process, helping us to systematically refine our thinking about policies, potentially even before they have been implemented in the real world.

While models are therefore useful for addressing public health policy questions, few consumers of models will comb through all of a model's detailed equations to fully analyze the complex relationships embedded in a given model. How does a modeler choose to represent a disease or public health program in a model, and how do we know whether to trust this representation? As we will illustrate, simply determining whether a model structure appears "realistic" can be misleading. Furthermore, looking at the list of assumptions that went into a given model is also insufficient to answer this model choice question. Counterintuitively, some models with many simplifying assumptions may actually be more helpful to answer key policy questions than more complex models, as we will illustrate.

MODELS ARE BECOMING MORE COMPLEX, PRESENTING NEW CHALLENGES TO READERS

It is rarely the case that one model is obviously "superior" to others for modeling a given policy problem. There are many ways to represent the pathogenesis of a given disease, even one that is well characterized. Alternative models have been constructed to simulate the same policy problem, using the same information. For example, very different models were recently used to simulate the reduction of transmission of human immunodeficiency virus (HIV) due to antiretroviral treatment and to simulate the cholera epidemic in Haiti, with differing results.[1-4] How can readers compare and contrast the results of these models?

Most readers will recognize that reviewing a model's assumptions is an essential component to answering whether a model might apply to a given scientific question—especially if assumptions strongly contradict available data or if the assumptions render the model inapplicable to a given policy environment. But a drive to make models more "realistic" has led to increasingly complex models with high levels of detail.[5]

The trend toward increasing complexity may allow scientists to address increasingly subtle or complex dimensions of a policy problem but also poses several potential challenges. First, readers should be aware that increasing the number of variables, or parameters, in a model can produce unintended effects. As shown in Figures 11.1 and 11.2, the number of factors that are included in a model does not determine how well it will forecast a particular outcome, such as a disease prevalence rate or a cost-effectiveness ratio. Rather, every additional parameter in the model introduces new sources of uncertainty and potential to affect results in nonintuitive ways that may either be useful (the model helps identify a critical issue) or deceptive

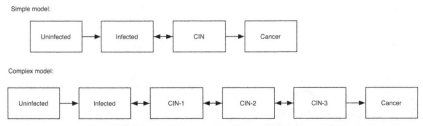

FIGURE 11.1 Two alternative models of human papillomavirus and cervical cancer. Precancerous states are designated as cervical intraepithelial neoplasia (CIN) stages 1, 2, and 3.

(the model produces strange behavior that reflects the model structure, not a true aspect of disease pathogenesis).

Figure 11.1 provides a comparison of two SIR-type simulation models that were extended to simulate the transmission of human papillomavirus and subsequent incidence of cervical cancer. The models were used to first generate data describing the prevalence of all cervical intraepithelial neoplasia (CIN) lesions, which are precancerous lesions, over a 30-year period among a cohort of young women. The more complex of the two models includes multiple latent states of illness (multiple stages of precancerous lesions), which can progress or regress at rates that are poorly characterized. This more complex model may seem more "realistic". But to illustrate the danger of favoring the more complex models, we used typical parameter values for the rates of progression and regression between states (a 5% rate of progression to the next state and 50% rate of regression per year to the prior state), then added noise to the data by drawing randomly from a normal distribution with mean equal to average prevalence and standard deviation corresponding to the prevalence rate's standard deviation. We performed a common model "calibration" approach in which both the simple and complex models shown in Figure 11.1 were fitted to the first 20 years of the data (solid dots), starting from standard parameter uncertainty ranges for progression and regression of disease.[6]

In Figure 11.2, we see an illustration of the danger of fitting the more complex model to limited data. Despite being a more "realistic" model, the more complex model had numerous alternative parameter values fit the data because there are so many uncertainties about the progression and regression rates that many combinations of parameters were able to produce reasonable fits. As shown, one of these fits produced a pattern that poorly forecast future prevalence (hollow dots) despite fitting the earlier prevalence data (solid dots). The more complex model actually has a better "fit" to the early prevalence data when judged by standard reduced chi-squared criteria than does the simpler model; but, as illustrated here, it has substantially poorer performance in forecasting prevalence in future years. The more complex model did not perform poorly simply by chance; it did so because there was

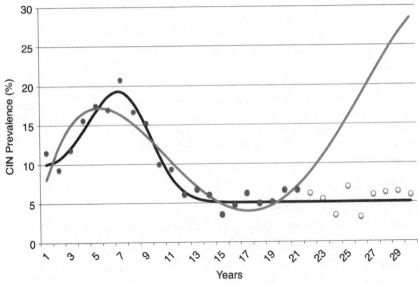

FIGURE 11.2 An illustration of the danger of overfitting a model to data in a theoretical demonstration. We first generated data describing the prevalence of all cervical intraepithelial neoplasia (CIN) lesions over a 30-year period among a fictional cohort of young women. To do so, we used the more "realistic" (complex) model in Figure 11.1 and assigned typical parameter values for the rates of progression and regression between states (a 5% rate of progression to the next state and 50% rate of regression per year to the prior state), then added noise to the data by drawing randomly from a normal distribution with mean equal to average prevalence and standard deviation corresponding to the prevalence rate's standard deviation. We performed a common model "calibration" approach in which both the simple and complex model shown in Figure 11.1 were fitted to the first 20 years of the data (solid dots), starting from standard parameter uncertainty ranges for progression and regression of disease. Despite being the "real" model, the more complex model had numerous alternative parameter values fit the data, since there are so many uncertainties about the progression and regression rates that many combinations of parameters were able to produce reasonable fits. As shown, one of these fits produced a pattern that poorly forecast future prevalence (hollow dots) despite fitting the earlier prevalence data (solid dots). The more complex model (wavy line) actually has a better "fit" to the early prevalence data when judged by standard reduced chi-squared criteria than does the simpler model (less wavy line); but as illustrated here, it has substantially poorer performance in forecasting prevalence in future years. The more complex model did not perform poorly simply by chance; it did so because there was insufficient prior knowledge to inform the parameter values describing the process of progression and regression through pre-cancerous states, hence the model was susceptible to fitting too tightly to the noisy prevalence data (overfitting).

insufficient prior knowledge to inform the parameter values describing the process of progression and regression through precancerous states; hence, the model was susceptible to fitting too tightly to the noisy prevalence data (overfitting). This outcome reveals that complex models must be well-characterized in terms of their behavior before they are used for forecasting or the simulation of disease interventions.

DILEMMAS OF MODEL "CALIBRATION"
AND "VALIDATION"

Whereas Figure 11.2 illustrates the irony that adding more variables to a model may actually make a model less "realistic" if its parameters' values or behaviors are not well understood, it would seem that ensuring that a model "fits" external data should be a sufficient check on the model's validity. "Calibration" algorithms have been devised to fit large models to data, often allowing modelers to infer the value of parameters that are difficult, if not impossible, to observe in real-world studies.[7]

However, there are important limitations to model fitting that readers should be aware of. By varying more parameters to fit data, a more complex model can "overfit" the data—as illustrated in Figure 11.2; the more complex model in the figure fits the early prevalence data more tightly but "misses the forest for the trees" by failing to capture just those key aspects of disease pathogenesis that are most relevant to determining the overall prevalence of disease. This occurs because so many parameters can be varied over their range of uncertainty that their inferred or "fitted" values can become overly influenced by noise in the dataset, as illustrated graphically in Figure 11.2.

Rather than proving that a model is "valid," fitting a model to data should be thought of as a way to "screen out" a model. That is, if the model can't be fit to data using any reasonable ranges for the parameters, then either the model structure is a poor representation of the actual disease process, or the range of parameter values is far from their real-world values. But fitting is not "proof" that a model is the "correct" one since there are many models that can reasonably fit the same set of external data.[8]

A more difficult problem with fitting models is the issue of "identifiability": when a large number of model parameters are being fit to a small number of data points, multiple different values can be assigned to each variable. More complex models will almost always fit external data more closely; more variables mean more degrees of freedom—more "wiggle room" among parameter values—to fit external data. Far from improving a model, calibrating too many parameters to too little data can produce several inaccuracies.

AN EXAMPLE OF THE IDENTIFIABILITY PROBLEM

To illustrate the identifiability problem, consider the following model of HIV. A principal concern is how much transmission occurs during the period of acute HIV infection, before an individual can be detected by standard diagnostic tests.[9,10] Suppose we have a model of HIV with just two parameters: the number of infections per month during acute HIV infection and the duration of elevated transmission risk during acute infection. But we only have one data point that tells us that a typical infected person causes six secondary infections during their acute infectious period. The rate of generating infections and the duration of acute disease can be varied over many values to fit this single data point; for instance, the rate of infection might be six per month, and the duration of acute disease 1 month, or 3 and 2, or 1 and 6, respectively, all of which multiply to the same number of secondary infections. This is what is meant by a *nonidentifiable model*: multiple combinations of parameters can generate the same observed data, such that the true values of the parameters cannot be determined by the model and available data (Figure 11.3).

In Figure 11.3, both a 1-month duration of acute infection with six secondary infections per month (top graph) and a 3-month duration of acute infection with two secondary infections per month (bottom graph) produce the same result of six infections per person during the acute infectious period. But the implications of the two different parameter sets are very different because early treatment (red dashed line) would be effective in preventing secondary infections only in the latter case.

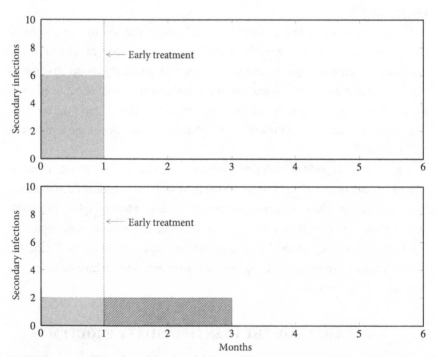

FIGURE 11.3 An illustration of the identifiability problem, using an example from HIV policy. Both a 1-month duration of acute infection with six secondary infections per month (top graph) and a 3-month duration of acute infection with two secondary infections per month (bottom graph) produce the same result of six infections per person during the acute infectious period. But the implications of the two different parameter sets are very different, as early treatment (dashed line) would be effective in preventing secondary infections only in the latter case.

If there were more data to triangulate the parameter values, then we would be able to solve this problem. But since all of these parameters fit equally well to our one data point, the average result from a calibration will simply be the midpoint of the range of parameter values that the modeler specified. For example, if a range of 1 to 5 months were chosen as possible values for the duration of acute infection, the average result would be 3 months at two infections/month. Suppose the true values for the parameters are duration of 1 month and six infections/month. If our model was simulating an intervention to treat acute HIV (e.g., the "test and treat" strategy of screening for acute infection and giving antiretroviral medications at 1 month into the infection[11] or behavioral interventions to reduce sexual risk upon diagnosis[12]), then the true impact on transmission during acute infection would be nil, while the model would project that four infections would be averted (2/month × (3 − 1) months) as shown in Figure 11.3.

Even computationally intensive "calibration" algorithms that search for millions of possible parameter values to fit a dataset can't overcome the identifiability problem. Because there is not sufficient information to tell which parameter values are more likely to be accurate than others, averaging the results of multiple fits will not work, and sensitivity analyses will be sampling from an infinite range of possibilities (an uninformative result). Many parameters' values can all be fit to data reasonably well, but the mean (or median) of the results will typically be a poor descriptor of the actual parameter space.[13] The recommended approaches to remedy a failure of identifiability are to (a) return to the field and gather more data to inform the parameter values in the model, (b) use a simpler model that requires fewer parameters if possible, or (c) conduct a theoretical analysis that explores various alternative parameter sets and their potentially different outcomes.

SENSITIVITY, UNCERTAINTY, AND MODEL SELECTION APPROACHES

When faced with so many uncertainties about the values of parameters and even the structure of models being used to simulate disease, it is common for modeling papers to include sensitivity analyses in which the value of each parameter is varied across its range of possible values. This helps to examine how raising or lowering a parameter's value may raise or lower the value of a model's outcome variable. Similarly, "uncertainty analysis" involves generating error bars around the model's results by sampling from the probability distributions describing the parameter values, examining how variations in the parameter values result in uncertainty around the model's results.[14]

However, a common mistake is to assume that sensitivity and uncertainty analyses capture the possible range of results that might occur in the real world. Typical sensitivity and uncertainty analyses involve varying a model's parameter values, not varying the underlying model structure (i.e., the way of representing a disease). Hence, "parameter uncertainty" is captured, but not "structural uncertainty." Differences in how models are structured can have a greater impact on model projections than differences in parameter values.[15] Variations in the value of a given parameter value could result in a markedly different range of results when that same parameter is input into a different model structure.[16]

To address this dilemma, a number of new strategies have been created to perform explicit "model selection"—that is, to generate several alternative model structures and use objective criteria to evaluate which models can best balance complexity and uncertainty (maximizing fit with the fewest parameters to minimize error). These range from likelihood-based methods that express the probability of the observed data under a particular model, to Bayesian methods that can avoid the complexities of computing a likelihood function for a complex model (such as Markov chain Monte Carlo methods that select not only parameter values but also "jump" between alternative model structures).[17,18] The strategies all follow one basic principle: that data should inform the level of complexity in a model.

If a particular model structure is too simple to address the research question under consideration, then critical variables can be added or alternative model structures chosen so that the disease can be simulated with an appropriately higher degree of complexity. Conversely, if a proposed model is too complex to properly estimate its unknown parameters as relevant to the dataset being used, then the selection method identifies that model as problematic and favors a simpler model. In some instances, a modeler may choose the more complex model because of strong a priori beliefs about the necessity of capturing a certain disease or policy process or the finding that a complexity can alter the results in critically informative ways (i.e., the complexity is critical to the question being asked—e.g., in the case of a sexually transmitted disease, the sexual network structure may be critical to ask questions about how heterogeneous contact patterns may influence transmission). In such instances, it should be possible to justify why a more complex model is being utilized. Recent reviews, however, have found that several models can often be employed for the same policy question using the same data[15,19]; hence, an obviously "optimal" model for a given policy problem may be a rare finding.

To date, selection algorithms have only rarely been used in the medical and public health literature[8] and have not been incorporated into guidelines for model reporting,[20,21] even though the approaches have been extensively researched and in some cases automated. While it is much faster to generate one model structure than to undertake the task of comparing alternative models formally, performing explicit model comparisons and selection may be critical to assessing the "robustness" of public health policy modeling results in the future. This would be analogous to the selection of individuals in clinical trials: we require prespecified, objective criteria for investigators to choose study participants; hence, prespecified, objective criteria can similarly be applied to policy model selection.

CONCLUSION

Modelers are usually asked by reviewers and readers to defend simplifying assumptions in models; it would also be reasonable, given the issues discussed here, for reviewers and readers to ask modelers to justify "nonessential complexity" with equal vigor. Models can be treated like computational versions of laboratory experiments—they are meant to explicitly highlight the assumptions that are implicit in health policy proposals, setting up a "clean" analysis to characterize and understand the relationships between key factors affecting health outcomes. Models should, as with laboratory experiments, be sufficiently transparent that their results can be replicated. Models serve as useful tools even when they are simple representations of the real world; new techniques can help us find the right balance between parsimony and realism in an objective manner, using data to build the model from the best available information for any given policy question. As Albert Einstein stated: "Everything should be made as simple as possible, but not simpler."

REFERENCES

Introduction

1. King G. Charles Proteus Steinmetz, the Wizard of Schenectady. Smithsonian. [Cited August 3, 2016.] Available from: http://www.smithsonianmag.com/history/charles-proteus-steinmetz-the-wizard-of-schenectady-51912022/
2. US Centers for Disease Control and Prevention. *2014 Ebola Outbreak in West Africa - Case Counts*. Atlanta: CDC, 2014.
3. Andrews JR, Basu S. Transmission dynamics and control of cholera in Haiti: an epidemic model. *Lancet*. 2011 Apr 9;377(9773):1248–55.

Chapter 1

1. Kron J. In Uganda, an AIDS success story comes undone. *N Y Times*. 2 August 2012.
2. Slater CA, Davis RB, Shmerling RH. Antinuclear antibody testing. A study of clinical utility. *Arch Intern Med*. 1996;156:1421–5.
3. Aschengrau A, Seage GR. *Essentials of Epidemiology in Public Health*. Burlington, MA: Jones & Bartlett Publishers, 2013.
4. Leung CW, Villamor E. Is participation in food and income assistance programmes associated with obesity in California adults? Results from a state-wide survey. *Public Health Nutr*. 2011;14:645–52.
5. Almada L, McCarthy IM, Tchernis R. *What Can We Learn About the Effects of Food Stamps on Obesity in the Presence of Misreporting?* National Bureau of Economic Research, 2015.
6. Buffler PA, Ginevan ME, Mandel JS et al. The Air Force health study: an epidemiologic retrospective. *Ann Epidemiol*. 2011;21:673–87.
7. Mitchell AA, Cottler LB, Shapiro S. Effect of questionnaire design on recall of drug exposure in pregnancy. *Am J Epidemiol*. 1986;123:670–6.

Chapter 2

1. Klarman HE, Rosenthal GD. Cost effectiveness analysis applied to the treatment of chronic renal disease. *Med Care* 1968;6:48–54.
2. Torrance GW. Measurement of health state utilities for economic appraisal. *J Health Econ* 1986;5:1–30.
3. Grosse SD. Assessing cost-effectiveness in healthcare: history of the $50,000 per QALY threshold. 2008.
4. Pruss-Ustun, A., Mathers, C., Corvalan, C., Woodward, A. Introduction and methods: Assessing the environmental burden of disease at national and local levels. Geneva: World Health Organization, 2003.

5. World Health Organization. Disability weights, discounting and age weighting of DALYs. Geneva: WHO, 2017.
6. Katz DA, Welch HG. Discounting in cost-effectiveness analysis of healthcare programmes. *PharmacoEconomics* 1993;3:276–85.

Chapter 3

1. Arora RK. *Optimization: Algorithms and Applications.* 1st edition. Boca Raton: Chapman and Hall/CRC, 2015.

Chapter 6

1. Bailey R. Growing a better future: food justice in a resource-constrained world. *Oxfam Policy and Practice: Agriculture, Food and Land.* 2011;11:93–168.

Chapter 8

1. Norton JA, Bass FM. A diffusion theory model of adoption and substitution for successive generations of high-technology products. *Mgmt Sci.* 1987;33:1069–86.
2. Schelling TC. Models of segregation. *Am Econ Rev.* 1969;59:488–93.
3. Müller B, Bohn F, Dreßler G et al. Describing human decisions in agent-based models–ODD+ D, an extension of the ODD protocol. *Environm Model Softw.* 2013;48:37–48.

Chapter 10

1. Heffernan J, Smith R, Wahl L. Perspectives on the basic reproductive ratio. *J R Soc Interface.* 2005;2:281–93.

Chapter 11

1. Eaton JW, Johnson LF, Salomon JA et al. HIV treatment as prevention: systematic comparison of mathematical models of the potential impact of antiretroviral therapy on HIV incidence in South Africa. *PLoS Med.* 2012;9:e1001245.
2. Andrews JR, Basu S. Transmission dynamics and control of cholera in Haiti: an epidemic model. *Lancet.* 2011;377:1248–55.
3. Rinaldo A, Blokesh M, Beruzzo E et al. A transmission model of the 2010 cholera epidemic in Haiti. *Ann Intern Med.* 2011;155:403–4.
4. Tuite AR, Tien J, Eisenberg M et al. Cholera epidemic in Haiti, 2010: using a transmission model to explain spatial spread of disease and identify optimal control interventions. *Ann Intern Med.* 2011;154:593–601.
5. May RM. Uses and abuses of mathematics in biology. *Science.* 2004;303:790–3.
6. Basu S, Chapman GB, Galvani AP. Integrating epidemiology, psychology, and economics to achieve HPV vaccination targets. *Proc Natl Acad Sci.* 2008;105:19018–23.
7. Basu S, Galvani AP. Re: "Multiparameter calibration of a natural history model of cervical cancer." *Am J Epidemiol.* 2007;166:983–983.
8. Basu S, Stuckler D, Bitton A et al. Projected effects of tobacco smoking on worldwide tuberculosis control: mathematical modelling analysis. *BMJ.* 2011;343:d5506.

9. Pinkerton SD. Probability of HIV transmission during acute infection in Rakai, Uganda. *AIDS Behav.* 2008;12:677–84.

10. Pilcher CD, Christopoulos KA, Golden M. Public health rationale for rapid nucleic acid or p24 antigen tests for HIV. *J Infect Dis.* 2010;201:S7–15.

11. Powers KA, Ghani AC, Miller WC et al. The role of acute and early HIV infection in the spread of HIV and implications for transmission prevention strategies in Lilongwe, Malawi: a modelling study. *Lancet.* 2011;378:256–68.

12. Steward WT, Remien RH, Higgins JA et al. Behavior change following diagnosis with acute/early HIV infection—a move to serosorting with other HIV-infected individuals. The NIMH Multisite Acute HIV Infection Study: III. *AIDS Behav.* 2009;13:1054–60.

13. Bolker BM. *Ecological Models and Data in R.* Princeton: Princeton University Press, 2008.

14. Blower SM, Dowlatabadi H. Sensitivity and uncertainty analysis of complex models of disease transmission: an HIV model, as an example. *Intl Stat Rev/Revue Internationale de Statistique.* 1994:229–43.

15. Suthar AB, Lawn SD, del Amo J et al. Antiretroviral therapy for prevention of tuberculosis in adults with HIV: a systematic review and meta-analysis. *PLoS Med.* 2012;9:e1001270.

16. Andrews JR, Wood R, Bekker L-G et al. Projecting the benefits of antiretroviral therapy for HIV prevention: the impact of population mobility and linkage to care. *J Infect Dis.* 2012;206:543–51.

17. Toni T, Welch D, Strelkowa N et al. Approximate Bayesian computation scheme for parameter inference and model selection in dynamical systems. *J R Soc Interface.* 2009;6:187–202.

18. Bortz D, Nelson P. Model selection and mixed-effects modeling of HIV infection dynamics. *Bull Math Biol.* 2006;68:2005–25.

19. Eyles H, Mhurchu CN, Nghiem N et al. Food pricing strategies, population diets, and non-communicable disease: a systematic review of simulation studies. *PLoS Med.* 2012;9:e1001353.

20. Rahmandad H, Sterman JD. Reporting guidelines for simulation-based research in social sciences. *Syst Dynam Rev.* 2012;28:396–411.

21. Grimm V, Berger U, DeAngelis DL et al. The ODD protocol: a review and first update. *Ecologic Model.* 2010;221:2760–8.

INDEX